The PCOS Environmental Roadmap

Dian Ginsberg, MD
with
Sheila Vuckovic, M.Ed., NTP

This book is not intended as a substitute for the medical advice of physicians. The reader should regularly consult a physician in matters relating to his or her health and particularly with respect to any symptoms that may require diagnosis or medical attention. Any eating or lifestyle change should be undertaken only under the direct supervision of the reader's personal physician. The reader should not stop any prescription medications without the consent of his or her personal physician. Readers with chronic health conditions, or who are pregnant or nursing, should not undertake any of the advice in this book without first checking with their own personal physician.

This book is dedicated to those who have suffered with Polycystic Ovarian Syndrome. You inspire us every day to make the world a better place.

Introduction

Who could have guessed that my two sons with dyslexia would lead me down the path to write a book on PCOS or polycystic ovarian syndrome? Although seemingly unconnected, this pathway will seem inevitable once you read my story.

The issues my boys were facing and their subsequent treatment protocols influenced my medical practice as a young OB/GYN physician to start thinking outside the box. I thought, instead of using birth control pills as Band-Aids for issues such as PCOS, what if I took a different approach? The greatest upsets in history came from those who thought a bit more originally, like the Wright Brothers or Henry Ford, and I realized if I wanted to change the world for my sons, I could start with how I practice medicine.

Andy, my oldest son, was born at term in an uncomplicated vaginal delivery. Douglas followed three and a half years later. While all their physical milestones were reached on time, Andy did not say "mommy" and had what seemed like no understandable language until three and a half years old. I thought that was an isolated incident until Doug's first word did not come until just before he turned five. We took him to countless specialists when there were no words after his second birthday, and I was told he might never speak! When he finally did speak that first word, it was not an instant recovery. The language and learning process occurred slowly, and I was becoming disheartened with the traditional methods offered by the experts.

Meanwhile at my OB/GYN practice, I started to notice more and more patients complaining about fatigue, weight gain, hormone imbalance, and premenstrual syndrome or PMS. I had been in practice for ten years at this time, and things seemed to be rapidly changing for my patients. I began to see huge increases in young females presenting with complaints similar to the above, along with irregular menses, acne, and infertility. These patients all met the criteria for a PCOS diagnosis, and the supported "treatment" for it was birth control pills.

I remember attending a medical conference around that time and hearing an older endocrinologist state that when she was in residency, she was told that she would see maybe two patients with PCOS in a lifetime. Now she was seeing one to two per week. In my present office practice, we often see two per day.

So how do the learning differences in my boys relate to my approaching PCOS in a new light? The thought processes are the same. The body is a perfect machine, and if it is not functioning optimally, we need to find out why and discover what went wrong to try to correct it.

With my boys, I went back to the roots of who they are. That would be their gut and their microbiome on the inside and the environment in which they were living on the outside. Thus began the change in the way we lived our life. The whole foods we ate and the amount and variation of plants and vegetables we consumed increased. The amount of computer and video exposure was limited, sunshine and circadian rhythms were respected, and we looked at nutrient deficiencies and supplemented what was needed. Language and learning in both boys dramatically increased. Eventually I was told they had a "processing issue" where they processed and comprehended words through their brains differently. This was a dramatically different label than we had received before and brought me hope. To this day, as adults, they think differently—but is that not a good thing? Different is good and can move mountains.

This is what I also started to see in my office. When taking the PCOS diagnosis and looking at the world in which the patient was living, it was clear that often the internal gut and external environment were the pathway that led to the development of the syndrome. If these young women kept on that same path and were simply given pills, just as I had been told to do with my boys, they would wind up at a frustrating dead end. I decided to take what I had learned and make a difference.

Learning of the functional medicine approach to health, I was completely convinced this concept was the solution. The answer was not in giving a pill but in diving into the root cause. Adding all the supplementary support in micronutrient deficiencies, inflammation healing, digestion and gut bacteria balancing, minimizing free radical effects, and reconnecting to our circadian rhythms in our environment produced excellent results in our office practice. Reversal of PCOS with healthy weight, normalized menses, renewed energy, and the ability to conceive were common occurrences.

When my youngest son was five years old, I was told he had an IQ of 50 and would never speak. Today he is a college student at Southwestern University, doing very well academically and running both track and cross country. You hold your future in your hands and have the ability to travel down any road you choose. While I have delivered over ten thousand babies in my career, my passion now is helping those "babies" who are now grown find the real path to health. I hope you approach this book with the same passion with which I wrote it.

In wellness,

Dian Ginsberg, MD

Table of Contents

List of Figures

List of Tables

Chapter 1. Myth Busting: A New Light

"Life is like riding a bicycle. To keep your balance,
you must keep moving."
Albert Einstein

The menstrual cycle is one of the most beautiful and mysterious processes. How amazing that the female body responds and synchronizes to the circadian rhythm of the earth! What a great signal we as women receive every month when that 28- to 32-day cycle occurs regularly that all is well within the body. However, for many women, the menstrual cycle is dreaded every month for occurring too early and too often, for causing pain and mood swings, or for simply ceasing to come at all. We have found that many women have no idea what is really happening inside their body and don't really understand what it means to truly have hormonal balance.

Excess hair growth, acne, irregular and/or absent periods, and infertility have been among the most common reasons women visit our practice in Houston, Texas. Each of these symptoms appears to come out of nowhere and slowly creep into their lives like a dark shadow. They often only find themselves in our hybrid OB/GYN–Functional Medicine office as a last resort, after their daily existence became overwhelmed by the constant search for answers in countless doctors' offices, online, or from well-meaning friends and family.

Once the diagnosis of PCOS (polycystic ovarian syndrome) is given, instead of clarity, even more confusion and frustration arise. What exactly does that mean? The words "you have PCOS," usually come along with a pack of birth control pills and a recommendation to eat better and exercise. While birth control pills may be needed as a *temporary* solution for heavy bleeding in certain patients, these pills are far from a cure. Many women whose monthly cycles return to normal on the birth control pill truly think their irregular menses and PCOS are cured (and many doctors never tell them otherwise). They unfortunately find a different story when they stop the pill and try to get pregnant.

This brings up a different question: What really is this PCOS and can it be *cured*? Even more important: Is it really a *sickness* that is *cured* with a medication?

If you are reading this book, thank you for trusting us on your path as you search for answers. While there are many books on PCOS to read, the journey revealed in this book is different. We must look at PCOS not as a medical sickness to be diagnosed and cured, but as a state of being that developed based on our genetics, activity, and complete internal and external environments.

Mother Nature is absolutely brilliant, and she has brought us life and adaptation to enable survival for billions of years. She has equipped the female body in all species to live and procreate even when food is scarce for months. Energy to live comes not only from the organic food we consume but also from the light we extract from the sun and our outdoor surroundings. Even in our modern world, all species still respect seasonal changes in food, activity, and circadian rhythm (light/dark cycle).

However, sometimes we tend to take this innate intelligence for granted and try to outsmart Mother Nature. When we look at our modern-day life, much of those "rhythms of life" are disrupted. The electrical and magnetic forces that surround us every day to ensure the perfect energy balance in tune with the environment have been disrupted by not only our food abundance and quality but also our lack of light and the inundation of technology's electro-smog. This electro-smog is the excess invisible electromagnetic radiation that results from the excess use of all our wireless technology. The woman who has lost her connection with her ancestral genetic predisposition and the rhythm of her environment will experience a state of dysregulation. This dysregulation may manifest as PCOS in the genetically susceptible female.

Once you understand a bit of how women evolved, we will give you a roadmap to help you regain your health and vitality. We will discuss the symptoms of PCOS and how the medical community defines it, but more important, give you an understanding of its development. Understanding gives you the power to take your life back to the healthy place you were meant to be.

The journey to hormonal balance and freedom from PCOS dysregulation requires navigating *The PCOS Environmental Roadmap.* It actually begins by stepping outside your body cells into your environment. How you interact with your surroundings can create changes in your genes and body processes that can cause PCOS to manifest.

There are two environments that you interact with daily. The first environment is the one you visualize every day. The earth and the sunlight we absorb daily, both visually and through our skin, have been instrumental in human development for as long as we have been on this planet. It is through understanding, respect, and interaction with our environment that we grow, live, and reproduce. Modern day has forgotten this concept. Lack of sunlight, increase in blue light, loss of seasonal rotation of both food and activities, and electromagnetic fields from our cell phones and other technologies have disrupted our circadian rhythms. *Circadian rhythm* refers to the "sync" of our bodies with night/day and sleep/wake clocks and is one of the principal regulators of the female cycle. Dysregulation of these external forces can add to the development of PCOS.

The second environment is your gastrointestinal tract, also known as your gut. Your inside environment contains trillions of microbes that we call the microbiome. There is a lot of scientific study today about the microbiome and whether it is it part of your surroundings or actually part of you. You have more microbe or "bug" genes than your own genes, and many of these bugs spend large amounts of time in your intestines. They extract nutrients for you to use to make energy, and they make many of your essential vitamins necessary to live. They make the fatty acids that serve as the building blocks of your intestinal lining where they are essentially building and repairing their own "house" daily. Some are transient and are just passing through. Every day, you have an environment that passes through your body and dramatically affects you even though you cannot see it.

Because this inside environment is unseen, the impact is often not acknowledged and may be neglected. This relationship is one that we call *symbiotic*, meaning we take care of the microbes and they take care of us. If that relationship pact is broken, then consequences can occur.

If we strive for a true state of well-being, with respect for our feelings, bodies, and entire existence, then the various aspects of our every experience—be it physical, emotional, or environmental—will respond so as not to create an environment of disease, but instead one of strong body systems and increased health. Therefore, we have created a systemic approach to achieve this goal of true well-being. The PCOS Environmental Roadmap is divided into six parallel lanes that can and need to be traveled simultaneously:

1. **Energy balance**—including caloric intake and burn and movement beyond exercise (although that is also important)
2. **Genetics and epigenetics**—who we start as and who we become
3. **Microbiome**—our interactions with our internal environment
4. **Light**—our circadian rhythms and sunlight exposure (our interactions with the external environment)
5. **EMF**—electromagnetic force and its disruption of both our mitochondrial energy production and life's building blocks (external environment interacting with the internal)
6. **Hormone balance**—considering all hormones equally: estrogen and progesterone, as well as insulin, leptin, anti-Müllerian hormone, adiponectin, and all the thyroid hormones

This book is divided into multiple chapters, organized to take you on a journey through the development of PCOS. Each chapter illustrates specific areas of our body that have been affected along the way by the environment that surrounds us both inside and out. It presents scientific information through great practical examples and easily understood terms to help you understand why all the steps of the Roadmap must be followed to regain your health. We think you will find the science of PCOS understandable and fascinating. It will definitely instill a new respect for how amazing *every* female body is. The Roadmap illustrates the things you can initiate immediately and testing that you can ask for from your practitioner as you navigate back to health. We close out the book with a 28-Day PCOS Environmental Reset, designed to reset and synchronize your internal and external environments to put you on the road to recovery.

Chapter 2. Understanding the Diagnosis of PCOS and Why Birth Control Pills Are Not the Final Answer

"God gave us the gift of life; it is up to us to give ourselves the gift of living well."
Voltaire

We see a lot of confusion with our patients questioning if what they are experiencing is actually PCOS. Some patients have irregular cycles, while some do not. Some patients have hair growth and weight gain, while some do not. Maybe a doctor somewhere along their journey did a blood test and said they "could" have PCOS. These letters get assigned to women quite a bit in the medical community, and they are devastating and life changing. It helps to know what these letters and words mean to really understand the diagnosis. As you read further, you will learn that sometimes symptoms that seem like PCOS are actually caused by other body imbalances. Once the off-balance system is corrected, the symptoms disappear.

Polycystic means multiple cysts. *Ovarian* means on the ovaries. *Syndrome* is used because it's a collection of different symptoms that develop into a less than optimal state of being. There are generally three different clusters of symptoms that determine a PCOS diagnosis.

In 1990, the first international conference of PCOS was held at the National Institutes of Health. Based on a consensus survey of the attendees, instead of actual clinical data, the first diagnostic criteria for PCOS were proposed. In 2003, these criteria were expanded and became known as the Rotterdam criteria. The Rotterdam criteria require the presence of two of the following for an official PCOS diagnosis:

1. Chronic anovulation disorder (including oligo-ovulation: less than normal monthly ovulation; anovulation: lack of any ovulation; or amenorrhea: no menses at all);
2. Clinical acne, hirsutism (abnormal hair growth patterns), or biochemical signs of hyperandrogenism (too many male hormones); and

3. Presence of micro polycystic ovaries at ultrasound or presence of twelve or more follicles with a diameter of 2 ± 9 mm in each ovary, and/or increased ovarian volume (>10 mL)

In November 2015, the American Association of Clinical Endocrinologists (AACE), American College of Endocrinology (ACE), and Androgen Excess and PCOS Society (AES) released new guidelines in the evaluation and treatment of PCOS. While some changes were made and added, the Rotterdam trio is still the hallmark of the evaluation and diagnosis of PCOS.

Before we delve into what can go wrong, it is important to have some basic understanding of a normal system. Knowing about your endocrine system can really help as you take a look at the big picture of your internal and external environments and how you can use the Roadmap to help.

Normally, the female ovary releases an ova (oocyte) or "egg" once a month, signaling the body that it's time to have a baby. When that synchronization or communication of the central nervous system and the ovaries is ideal, the egg will be released about 2 weeks after the first day of your menstrual cycle. When no pregnancy occurs, your hormones drop, you shed your uterine lining, and you have a period. A normal cycle range is about 28–32 days. If you have a 34-day cycle one month and then a 26-day cycle the next month, and this happens irregularly, that is usually not a problem. It makes timing a pregnancy a bit more difficult, but bleeding cyclically somewhere in the mentioned range generally means you are ovulating.

On the other hand, if you don't have that normal cycle, then you aren't ovulating once a month, and we call that oligo-ovulation. *Oligo* means just a few or scant. Bleeding only every 3–4 months or every other month, bleeding at the beginning of one month and then again at the end of the next, spotting all the time, or bleeding every 2–3 weeks usually means you are not ovulating normally. This symptom is one of the criteria for a PCOS diagnosis.

Another factor for PCOS is a high level of androgens. Androgens are hormones that tend to be more male in nature. The most specific one that we see elevated in PCOS is testosterone. Testosterone can be either *total testosterone,* which is bound to other proteins, or *free testosterone,* which is unbound. Because free testosterone is not bound to other proteins, it is available in full to the tissues, therefore causing greater effects and unwanted symptoms like facial hair growth and acne in PCOS. Elevation of both free and total testosterone can develop as part of this syndrome, but elevated testosterone does not automatically mean you have PCOS. We will discuss more on this later in the book.

DHEA or dehydroepiandrosterone is another male hormone that is found in all women but is often elevated in women with PCOS. DHEA is secreted by the adrenal gland, but it is the hormone with the sulfur group attached that is measured in blood (DHEA-S). It is normal for women to have DHEA-S levels anywhere between 35 and 400 µg/dL. Most women with PCOS tend to have DHEA-S levels greater than 400 µg/dL. Levels even greater than this are a cause for concern and should be evaluated by an endocrinologist for the possibility of an adrenal tumor (although this is quite rare).

The third component—multiple cysts—is probably the most confusing. The development of an ovarian cyst seems to be easily misunderstood and misconstrued. Most women think *cyst* automatically means a pathological finding. Not true! Your ovary is actually about 3 cm around and has millions of pin head–size potential cysts, meaning potential spaces that can develop into a fluid-filled cavity or cyst.

Your central nervous system has to pick a follicle that contains a mature egg every month to get pregnant. The brain will send a stimulating hormone (follicle stimulating hormone or FSH) to integrate communication between itself and the ovary. Estrogen then rises and midcycle, about day 14, you ovulate (Figure 1). The cyst wall thins, and fluid within this mature oocyte is released into the fallopian tube to meet a sperm and form an early pregnancy. This happens in the context of a normal monthly cycle.

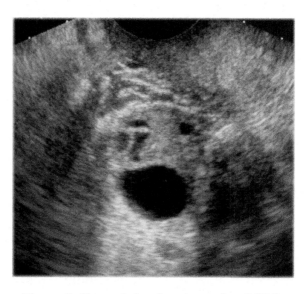

Figure 1. Normal dominant ovarian follicle

When ovulation occurs, your ovary has taken one of these potential little spaces and developed it into a single predominant cyst, the chosen one for the month. Along the way, many other little cysts develop. However, with the appropriate level of anti-Müllerian hormone (AMH) and overall hormone balance, on day 14 all the suboptimal cysts or follicles shrink while this predominate one lives. It then ovulates out the egg that is meant to become the pregnancy. It's very important to understand that the fluid-filled cyst cavity, called the *corpus luteum*, does not shrink and collapse immediately. Should you get pregnant, the corpus luteum secretes progesterone and keeps the fetus alive for three months until the placenta is mature and ready to do its job. If you don't get pregnant, the message is sent back that there's no baby this month. Therefore, hormones drop, the cyst dissolves, and you have a period. You can see the complexity of the integration between the central nervous system and your ovaries that has to happen in order to have a single cyst dominate and ovulate. You also see that the cyst is not this "bad thing" that women feel is plaguing them. It is only when the system is off that the cyst ruptures, gets too large, or twists on itself that a problem develops.

In PCOS, the dysfunction starts when a dominant follicle is never chosen. Instead of one follicle developing and ovulating, the complex hormonal cascade is dysregulated, the AMH is elevated, and a group of small cysts develop. This appears like a "string of pearls" on an ultrasound (Figure 2).

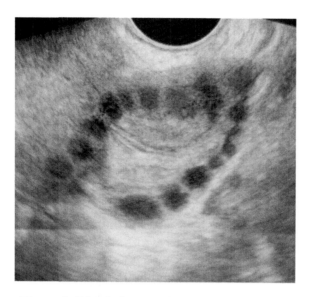

Figure 2. Multiple cysts in a polycystic ovary

Instead of that single, dominant cyst, this collection of confused little cysts grows, hence the multiple cysts in the Rotterdam criteria. *Again, you will make an ovarian cyst every month, and this process is normal.* Patients are often misinformed, believing that any type of ovarian cyst is a problem. It is important to remember that ovarian cysts develop monthly in the process of normal ovulation. But if the cyst overgrows, ruptures, or causes pain, that is a separate medical issue. In PCOS, however, the problem lies in the lack of the development of a dominant follicle or cyst.

Let us delve a little deeper into the development of the syndrome. PCOS occurs, in part, because of a dysfunctional signal between the ovaries and the central nervous system (CNS). Remember the old telephone game you played as a kid? One person spoke a message into another person's ear and the message was whispered down the line of friends. How clear the message was spoken and how carefully everyone listened determined whether the same message that started the game made it all the way to the end. A similar concept happens in the function of the human ovulation messaging system. Cells contain receptors on their membrane so they can receive hormone messages and pass them on to the DNA and other parts of the cell. When the receptor positioned in the cell membrane has the right genetics aligned with the right nutrients, environment, and activity, it can read the message appropriately. In PCOS, the message doesn't get read clearly, so the correct information is not entered into the cells of the ovary. Hormones such as testosterone and insulin are involved in this miscommunication. The ovarian receptor reads abnormal levels of insulin and testosterone, so the hormones released are not in the optimal balance for the brain to interpret and therefore create a normal cycle. Environmental factors such as imbalanced gut bacteria, imbalanced blood sugar, lack of sunlight, and increased electromagnetic field exposure all influence this communication. In later chapters, we will discuss in detail how you can keep your environment clean to encourage clear communication between the ovaries and the CNS.

As mentioned, birth control pills are the most prescribed "treatment" for PCOS. Please understand: These pills do *not* fix PCOS. Does birth control make you ovulate? It certainly makes it look like you are experiencing ovulation because these pills cause the shedding of the uterine lining, also known as your period. But the answer is a definite *no*!

Your uterus contains receptors that respond to estrogen and progesterone sent by the ovaries. The uterus creates a lining of blood in response to this estrogen, and progesterone follows to make a sort of "blanket" in the uterus to get ready for implantation. When the hormones decrease toward the end of your cycle, the blood vessels that feed the uterus fall and spiral away, causing the support blanket created by these hormones to fluff away. That's where the period comes from. This pattern is what the body naturally follows in a functional, natural cycle.

If you take the birth control pill, which contains estradiol (a type of estrogen) and progestin (a synthetic hormone that mimics progesterone but is in fact structurally different from your own progesterone), the uterus responds and makes blood. The amount and type of hormones in the pill influence the thickness of the uterine blood layer. That is, the thickness of the blanket of blood created in the uterus is influenced by the type of pill taken. Pills that contain very low amounts of estradiol cause the uterus to make even less blood, creating a very thin blanket. That's why low-dose birth controls pills may not cause withdrawal bleeding or a period at all. The pill has an end effect on the uterus but not the ovaries.

As explained previously, in PCOS the problem lies within the signaling and hormonal expression from the ovaries. Unfortunately, the estradiol/progestin combo doesn't change anything. *It just takes the ovaries out of the equation.* The uterus ignores everybody else, and it does what the pill tells it to do. Now when that woman who has had normal "birth control" cycles for years wants to get pregnant, she is often shocked that when she stops her birth control, she has abnormal cycles and infertility.

The pill also creates a false sense of security. All the symptoms of PCOS such as acne and irregular bleeding may decrease but the brain-ovarian hormonal balance is still not optimally functioning. Moreover, pills create inflammation and multiple nutrient deficiencies such as B6, B12, and folate. These side effects seem to be amplified in women with PCOS.

Metformin is another heavily prescribed medication for PCOS, second only to birth control pills. Many patients with PCOS are given metformin, an antidiabetic medication, because they are told that they have insulin resistance. However, it is interesting to note that the Rotterdam criteria do not list insulin resistance or blood sugar dysregulation as part of the criteria for diagnosis. Regulating blood sugar with dietary changes and/or medications such as metformin does seem to help normalize some patients with PCOS. We will get into the reason behind that, but our optimal goal is to help you understand your body and its relationship to the internal and external environment in order to stabilize your blood sugar and ovulate without medicine.

Remember, an optimal connection of the brain, environment, activity and nutrient status is ultimately what is needed to create hormonal harmony and health. These factors have also been found to influence changes in our DNA expression either directly or indirectly through what we call our *metabolic sensors*. These sensors have played an important role in human evolution, signaling the optimal times to eat, sleep, and procreate. They exist in our eyes when we see the morning sun and darkness of night, as well as in our cell nucleus to instruct our DNA in what proteins to order to be manufactured. We will dive into more detail on this little addressed topic and how it can make all the difference in reversing your PCOS.

It is so important to understand that if you take medication to alleviate your symptoms but not align yourself with all six lanes of the Roadmap, your outward *symptoms* may be alleviated, but the internal *dysfunction* will continue. While some medications can provide temporary relief, the goal of this book is to enable you to take control of your daily life and decrease, if not eliminate, the need for prescription medication. Of course, we do not recommend stopping anything without asking your physician. We also understand the need/want for some women to use a low-dose birth control pill to avoid pregnancy, which is why the birth control pill was created originally. Hopefully, this information will help you better partner with your health care provider to determine the best way to nourish your body in each stage of your life.

Chapter 3. Is PCOS Simply How We Survived as Cavewomen?

"While physics and mathematics may tell us how the universe began, they are not much use in predicting human behavior because there are far too many equations to solve. I'm no better than anyone else at understanding what makes people tick, particularly women."
Stephen Hawking

A true understanding of the ovaries and how evolution created these amazing machines will really help you on your journey. This tiny cluster of cells can change depending on the environment. In fact, the adaptability of the ovaries is integral to the continuation of the human race!

The following are questions we aim to answer for you in this chapter:

- Why isn't there a dominant follicle that takes over so I ovulate every month?
- What do those little cysts mean anyway?
- What is normal ovarian function, and what is dysfunction?
- Do genetics determine the function of the ovary and the ability to reproduce?
- If it is genetic, can it be changed?

Good news! Fate is not genetically predetermined because the environment plays a major role in determining how we progress through our health process. The stability lies in the system as a *whole*, not in individual genes. Much of who we are has to do with epigenetics or how genes *express* themselves. We may have the gene that says "do this," but how that trait is actually expressed or developed depends on a whole bunch of other things. You do have the power to change your health! Knowledge is truly powerful, so let's dive into the physiology and genetics of the ovary.

To review, there are a lot of little cysts normally contained in the ovary. These are microscopic and waiting to be picked as the dominant follicle to ovulate. When there is a dysregulation in the body, these little cysts grow a small amount and you will get the "string of pearls" you see on an ultrasound.

Here is where we dive just a bit deeper into the cells of the ovary. Your ovary is made up of millions of cells that all are connected together and cross talk. Surrounding the ovary is a surface made up of cells that have tiny receptors all over them. These surface receptors talk to the blood, other cells, and tissues that surround them. Cell receptors sit on the cell membrane and respond to chemical messages sent by the hormones. Hormones sail through your blood, sit on specific cell receptors, and send a message to the cell. Like two pieces of a puzzle, the fit between the hormone and the receptor needs to be perfect. If the match isn't perfect, the puzzle looks funny, meaning the hormone message won't be read correctly. It is extremely important that hormones and receptors match perfectly so they talk to each other efficiently. The right signal is given to the contents of the cell when that happens. While we are not exactly sure what is the issue in ovulation and the oocyte or egg quality in PCOS, science illustrates that the receptor and message transmission are part of the problem.

The adaptation that many PCOS patients have in their ovaries most likely served a very important purpose throughout evolution. Ovarian function relied on insulin and glucose balance to allow pregnancy to occur when food was plentiful, but shifted more to a fight-or-flight model in the dark, hungry months. Conservation of energy and timing of childbirth used to cycle around food availability, as still happens with animals today. The female reproductive system needs to be able to adapt to these changes. Our human environment, however, has changed very rapidly, and in today's society, "winter hunger" never comes. What was once very important for survival is no longer needed.

Research explains these changes in terms of the increasing development of PCOS. In the last few decades, we have learned that the B vitamin, inositol, can play a very important role in PCOS. Inositol exists in a variety of different shapes, but the two most important for proper ovarian function are the myo-inositol (MI) and the chiro-inositol (DCI) shape or isomer. Most MI is synthesized in the kidneys. It is converted to DCI in the ovaries (Figure 3). This conversion is affected by the amount of circulating insulin.

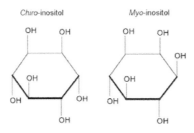

Figure 3. Structural differences of myo- and chiro-inositol

New research shows that the inositol isomers seem to be instrumental in controlling how glucose is utilized in cells. This emerging research supports the idea that the ideally balanced ratio of the two main inositol isomers, MI and DCI, control insulin signaling. MI is converted into DCI by the enzyme epimerase. When this enzyme is environmentally and/or genetically affected, the correct use of glucose and/or its storage as glycogen is disrupted. This would have been a protective mechanism during times of food scarcity.

When the ratio of these two inositol isomers is appropriately balanced and blood sugar and insulin within the body are balanced, one could say the overall female endocrine system is ready to reproduce. Insulin is a hormone that helps the body regulate the amount of glucose (sugar) in the blood. The greater the amount of glucose in the blood, the greater the amount of insulin required to bring the glucose level in the blood back to normal. Insulin is a life-giving hormone; without it, the cells are unable to be nourished. *It is the balance of this glucose in the ovarian cells and the blood that is important.* The ovaries contain insulin receptors because they also require this nourishment to function. They need to know if there is enough food to nourish a potential pregnancy. Just about every animal has to judge its environmental surroundings to ensure survival of the pregnancy and therefore the species. If there is too much glucose and insulin in the blood, the cells simply will not take in any more. That is what we call insulin resistance.

Sunny weather and plentiful food had paleolithic women eating and gaining weight seasonally to prep for winter. At the ovary, massive amounts of insulin begin "pounding" on the receptors to balance the glucose that is being consumed. As the environmental changes of glucose and insulin occurred in the cavewoman's body, insulin resistance occurred and the balance of the inositol isomers in the ovary changed. Less MI is converted to DCI, and small cysts that produce testosterone for the hard winter develop as opposed to the delicate follicle to become pregnant. It was a great survival tool.

Why would the body allow or even want changes in the ovary to cause the production of more testosterone? The animal kingdom provides some explanation, but to truly understand this concept, we need to understand the function of a very important protein called sex hormone binding globulin (SHBG). SHBG is a carrier protein produced by the liver that plays a critical role in regulating the amount of the unbound steroid hormones such as testosterone, dihydrotestosterone (DHT), and estrogen allowed to float freely in the blood. Hormones bound to this carrier protein are not available to tissues. Therefore, how much estrogen, testosterone, or other hormone is exposed to the cells depending on the environment can be controlled somewhat by this protein. SHBG also controls the flow of fatty acids throughout the body and is a type of back signal to the brain of the animal that its nutritional needs are met depending on the time of year.

Animals respect their circadian rhythms. This circadian rhythm tells them light and dark, warm and cold, summer and winter. Animals do not have houses or light bulbs or treadmills in the gym that they can run on at 8 pm after work. They sleep when it is dark and respect the sun when it is light. They collect food and put on weight in the summer so when winter arrives, they can survive on lean or no rations. However, even at its heaviest time, the bird can still fly south and the squirrel can still race up the tree. This feedback in the control of SHBG tells the animal when it has had enough to eat but still be lean enough to run for its life if necessary!

Low SHBG is an advantage to the animal in wintertime because it allows for higher amounts of free testosterone, hence more ability to be strong. If something attacks the animal during hibernation, they have enough testosterone to fight. This very important paleolithic or ancestral protective mechanism is what the cavewoman also used to survive hard times.

Now back to the importance of the MI/DCI conversion. If, as a cavewoman, your body was able to become insulin resistant and able to store glucose more easily than your neighbor, you would have a greater advantage when hard food times occurred unexpectedly. Even as recently in the last hundred years as the American West was conquered, strength through difficult food shortage and cold was optimal. It has been proposed that in women affected by PCOS, *ovaries remain insulin sensitive*, in contrast to most other tissues and organs such as muscle and liver, which can become insulin resistant. This probably served as an *advantage* during the hard winter months. The reproductive system knew when to work and when to rest.

Modern life has been around only as short as the blink of an eye. Therefore, these valuable traits that have kept us alive through starvation are still embedded in our genome, gut bacteria, or microbiome and overall who we are today. Society recently has changed fairly quickly in the abundance of food, heat, clothing, and shelter available. However, our cells are much slower at adapting to these changes.

Let us learn a bit about epimerase. The epimerase enzyme, located in the ovary, determines MI/DCI conversion and depends on the amount of insulin secreted into the blood. As would be expected, studies have shown there is a decreased amount of DCI production in insulin-sensitive tissues or organs such as the kidney, liver, and in the muscle of experimental animals with insulin resistance. However, an imbalance in MI conversion to DCI was seen not only in patients with type 2 diabetes but also in nondiabetic *relatives* of patients with diabetes. *Such data consistently supports the hypothesis that familial predisposition may induce an abnormal function/expression of epimerase enzyme activity.* Despite the fact that you may not have diabetes, your family lineage may pass on the abnormal enzyme function to you. You would then in any times of a more high glucose diet develop an MI/DCI imbalance, predisposing you to PCOS.

Other studies simply show that *the epimerase enzyme is just different in certain family lines.* We could speculate that PCOS patients with hyperinsulinemia (high insulin due to elevated glucose in the blood) likely present an abnormal MI to DCI conversion in the ovary. This overall imbalance could be responsible for the poor oocyte quality and infertility that occurs even with assisted reproductive techniques. We call it *unexplained infertility*. Rebalancing the myo/chiro-inositol ratio can help return the system to its optimal ovulating state.

What does all this mean? When we eat the nutrient-poor, processed, simple carbohydrates in our general diet today, the glucose and free fatty acids rise to extremely high levels. The body interprets that as the outside environment is summer and will begin to get ready for the famine of winter by increasing body fat and other hormones necessary to survive the scarcity of winter. *It will be more exaggerated if you genetically descend from a family whose body was very good at preparing for winter.* Unfortunately, in our present-day society, winter never comes. SHBG stays low indefinitely. In PCOS, this whole process is compounded. The extra testosterone that is produced by the ovary is left to float free by the constant low level of SHBG, leading to hair growth, acne, and all other symptoms that manifest when high testosterone persists. This is why it is helpful to have SHBG in the blood checked along with estradiol and total and free testosterone when trying to manage PCOS and its symptoms. It will give you an idea where you fit in this continuum.

In the next chapter, we will discuss insulin and how it can perpetuate the cycle just described. Chronic elevated insulin is an issue. However, what we are now also seeing is that the state of PCOS can reach such an extremely significant level of dysregulation that the body essentially gives up and can no longer manufacture insulin. *This can lead to the appearance of normal insulin levels in the blood.* This results in extreme frustration. The numbers look normal, so what is wrong? Why is the body not ovulating regularly or allowing for weight loss if everything is normal? The next chapter will delve further into the tricky world of insulin.

Chapter 4. The Real Deal on Insulin

"Life is 10% what happens to you and 90% how you react to it."
Charles R. Swindoll

The role of insulin in PCOS can really not be emphasized enough, so it will be discussed in even more detail in this chapter. Although the Rotterdam criteria have been widely accepted, it has recently become clear that a new clinical aspect needs to be taken into account: the dysregulation feature of insulin resistance. Indeed, if one does a deep literature search, insulin resistance is a frequent finding in patients with PCOS, regardless of body mass index (BMI). Chronically elevated insulin, as a result of dysregulated blood sugar, puts excessive stress on the endocrine system and can lead to the development of conditions such as PCOS. As this concept becomes clearer, the effect that your environment and lifestyle have on the manifestation of your genetics (epigenetics) will make more sense.

We understand that repetition of any new concept is always helpful in the learning process, so let's review the information we've discussed so far.

The cell membrane is the barrier between the proteins and other structures inside the cell and the bloodstream outside the cell. Receptors sitting on this cell membrane respond to hormones and their message. The hormone communicates the message to the hormone receptor on the cell membrane, then the cell performs whatever action was communicated. It is very similar to the lock-and-key metaphor, which many people are familiar with from Biology 101. If the key (the hormone) fits the lock (the receptor on the membrane) exactly, the message is communicated to the cell word for word. If the receptor is slightly altered because of some genetic mutations, the key fits not as perfectly and the message may not be received correctly by the cell. Higher levels of hormone must be released to try to have the message read.

Insulin is a very important hormone as it tells the cell when extra energy or glucose (sugar) is available and conveys that food is plentiful at this current time. Should there be a mutation of the receptor where the lock and key does not fit perfectly, then the cell will not understand or hear that it should store this glucose for the winter. The pancreas then releases more insulin since the glucose level in the blood remains elevated beyond what is ideal for the body.

Where hormones are concerned, insulin is the bully of the playground. If the blood level of glucose is constantly elevated, insulin will be called on in greater amounts to push the excess into the cells. Over time, it will be yelling at the cell to let more and more glucose in. However, the membrane knows that too much glucose in the cell is harmful. The cell membrane will eventually resist letting in any more glucose. The result is a toddler-like battle of wills: Insulin tells the cell to open up, and the cell resists, hence the term *insulin resistance.*

However, it was found out that the receptors on the ovary are actually *sensitive* to insulin; they do not develop insulin resistance. It is the other tissues in the body of a woman with PCOS that have trouble listening to the insulin message and develop this resistance. The muscle and fat tissues have slow glucose uptake and cause the disruptive insulin force to flow in excess all over the healthy tissues. It is the ovary that receives this extra insulin as it floats around the bloodstream, and the MCI/DCI conversion problem as described in the previous chapter develops. Hence, ovarian function and ovulation problems are created.

Having a healthy amount of muscle mass can help combat the development of insulin resistance. Therefore, regulating insulin levels by ensuring adequate muscle mass and appropriate effective exercise is a major part of the Roadmap back to health and balance.

If insulin levels remain stable, the genetic misalignment of the muscle insulin receptors leading to miscommunication of the hormones may be compensated for, and PCOS may not develop. This is the point of epigenetics—your genetic expression can be altered through the environment. Managing stress, eating a properly balanced, nutrient-dense diet, respecting circadian rhythms, obtaining restful sleep, controlling EMF (foreign electromagnetic fields) exposure, and proper exercise may keep dysregulation from developing. Problems occur when insulin is chronically high and upregulated due to constantly elevated blood glucose. This elevation is not always strictly diet related, but it is also affected by sleep, exercise, disruption of the light/dark cycles or circadian rhythm, and stress.

When you eat, blood glucose goes up, which is exactly what is intended in nature. This blood glucose is first sent to the brain and then to your muscles. Animals need and follow this same glucose-insulin balance. If the glucose in the bloodstream is still higher than the body finds comfortable after feeding the brain and muscles, it is sent to storage. Insulin carries this extra glucose to the liver cells first. The receptors on the cell membranes of the liver accept this message from insulin and store glucose in the form of glycogen in the liver. However, the liver cells only have small areas of storage, and the cell membrane will not allow any more glucose into these cells once they are full. Muscle cells will also take in glucose and store it as glycogen to be used to fuel exercise. This is another reason to continue to build and keep muscle mass for optimal female health.

If blood glucose is still elevated, insulin will turn to the fat cells for more storage. The fat cells have almost infinite space for storing glucose. Once the blood glucose is back down to levels that the body is comfortable with, insulin will stop communicating with the cells to try to push more glucose in. However, if the muscle and fat cells do not respond appropriately to the insulin message and glucose remains elevated, the brain signals to the pancreas to produce even more insulin.

Certain lifestyle choices along with this insulin receptor issue can lead to chronic insulin elevation. The signal of "all full, burn fat" can't be heard if insulin is constantly elevated. This puts the body in a perpetual state of panic that starvation is just around the corner. This state will prevent your body from ever getting to a point where it stops storing and becomes comfortable burning fat and losing weight. The message of balance does not come through clearly, so the body thinks that it constantly needs to store fat for emergencies instead of burning it.

It is in this situation that metformin is often prescribed: Metformin helps against high blood glucose. Its mode of action is mainly to decrease liver glucose production and increase the sensitivity of the body tissues to insulin. Interesting, the precise mechanism of action of metformin remains a bit unclear. Likely, it slows the use of glucose in the liver while acting on the membrane receptors of the muscle and fat cells. In plain speak, it makes the stubborn cells more sensitive to insulin.

Metformin, however, is a double-edged sword. In the case of developed insulin resistance, it will lower some of the blood insulin levels as the cells now uptake more. Decreasing glucose production may normalize your labs and make you look better on paper, but this is just a Band-Aid for PCOS. It is managing some of the symptoms but not addressing the root cause. If you keep flooding the system with nutrient-deficient foods high in simple carbohydrates and do not regain balance in your life, your system may eventually be overwhelmed. This is when the medical community starts to label you with illness such as unexplained infertility, cardiovascular disease, or diabetes. For some, metformin is simply not enough. This is why real lifestyle modifications through the PCOS Roadmap are necessary.

We will close this chapter by explaining the extreme importance of omega-3 fatty acids in insulin sensitivity. Omega-3 fatty acids are the very substance that increases the sensitivity to insulin by encouraging the cells to produce and secrete anti-inflammatory adiponectin while reducing the overall number of inflammatory and proinflammatory cells.

Adiponectin is secreted exclusively by mature fat cells and is one of the largest products of adipose/fat tissue. It is a fascinating hormone. Its circulating levels actually are reduced in obesity and insulin resistance, especially when fat accumulates around the waist. The newest research shows that adiponectin functions as an *insulin-sensitizing protein-hormone*. Adiponectin will keep the balance between the fat storage and burn while keeping the tissue insulin "sensitive." As you gain weight, adiponectin increases to keep inflammation and insulin effect in perfect balance. This sensitivity enables you to gain weight for the winter and mobilize the fat for energy when food sources disappear. This process all works fine until there becomes an unnatural scenario of too much fat accumulated and glucose intake still continues.

In wild animals, increased fat stores develop to get ready for winter hibernation. Those stored calories are burned during the winter famine, and the delicate balance continues. This is also how the human body has functioned for thousands of years until recently. Now in winter, we eat high-calorie holiday foods and have a continuous flow of calories. We gain weight around the waist to store for winter. However, "winter" (i.e., famine or even reduced flow of food) never comes. *Research has shown that as central body fat increases above what nature intended, we "break" this environmental cycle.*

Passing what is a balance intended for the body, adiponectin levels basically become overwhelmed and "give up." They now begin to decrease as midsection fat increases. As these levels drop, the kind work that adiponectin does to maintain insulin sensitivity disappears. In fact, the reduction in circulating adiponectin is considered as a mechanism whereby the process of developing obesity itself could cause the cascade of development of insulin resistance and diabetes. The vicious cycle keeps turning as the body becomes heavier and the adiponectin levels drop and the insulin resistance increases. Only by looking at the Roadmap lanes and controlling your environment can you restore your body's normal hormone levels.

Cognitive function and memory seem to also be affected by adiponectin levels, which is why this hormone is now being studied for antiaging benefits. Abnormal adiponectin levels have also been independently associated with memory loss. And given that glucose levels can affect adiponectin levels, it is not surprising that glucose regulation has been shown to have a significant impact on the maintenance of healthy thoughts and memory processing. When circulating at optimal levels, adiponectin exerts a wide range of beneficial effects on the cardiovascular and central nervous systems, having anti-inflammatory and antioxidant effects.

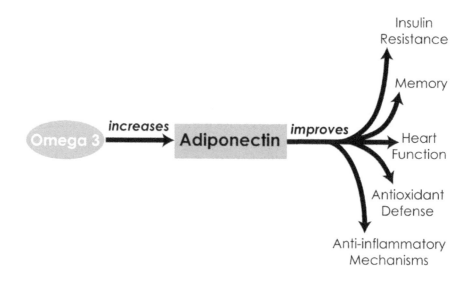

Figure 4. Effect of omega-3 on adiponectin

Insulin resistance is part of the underlying mechanism of PCOS. Adiponectin improves both insulin signaling and glucose uptake. Therefore, the takeaway message is that increasing adiponectin is part of an optimal pathway on the journey back to healthy weight and metabolism. Omega-3 fatty acids help increase adiponectin levels and therefore help restore insulin sensitivity. They can also reduce cholesterol absorption and synthesis, improve low-density lipoprotein (LDL) receptor activity in the liver, and increase LDL cholesterol breakdown. Instructions on how to test for healthy levels of omega-3 and adiponectin and how to improve these levels will be discussed in the Roadmap.

Chapter 5. Microbiome: Our Gut Rules Our Energy, Our Hormones, and So Much More!

"Am I simply a vehicle for numerous bacteria that inhabit my microbiome? Or are they hosting me?"
Timothy Morton

If you have spent any amount of time researching any health topic in the last few years, chances are the word *microbiome* has come up at some point. Although its origin in recent health literature is unclear (some publications state it didn't really come into fashion until 2001, others report it as early as the 1960s), the emerging research on this subject is fascinating. The communities of microorganisms that call us home are made up of more than one hundred trillion microbes and outnumber our human cells by a factor of 10. It's essentially their world, and they are just allowing us to live in it!

Our genetics are very simply not all our own. These microbial communities have a major impact on their host's (that's us!) health, metabolism, immunity, and hormones. These microbe colonies play a tremendous role in maintaining our vitality. The balance of these microbes is very important for optimal health. We are now learning that, should this delicate balance be disrupted, it exacerbates both genetic and environmental risks that lead to poor health outcomes.

The majority of these microbes live in our large intestine or gut. They make up our gut microbiome, which is made up of five hundred to a thousand different species that have a genome that collectively contains more genes than our own. This microbiome is now recognized as an "organ" in our body that actually performs functions. Digesting and processing food components, extracting calories, creating energy, and releasing toxins are only part of what this miraculous group of microorganisms can do. We are also learning that the gut microbiome determines what energy is stored, what is utilized, and how fat and glucose are managed. They also enable adequate nutrient breakdown and produce hormones, neurotransmitters (hormones that affect our central nervous system), vitamins, and healthy fats.

Internal balance within this microbiome is influenced dramatically by environmental effects. While working with us and attempting to optimize our health, our friendly "gut bugs" will change and dysregulate should they be exposed to less than optimal nutrients or inflammatory processed particles. Babies inherit their microbiome mostly from their mother, which is also influenced by the babies' mode of delivery into this world (C-section or vaginal birth) and first foods (breastfeeding, formula, etc.). These first factors, as well as other environmental and lifestyle factors throughout life, can alter the microbiome in a positive or negative way, leading to significant consequences and the extent to which PCOS develops.

Can a particular state of your microbial community predispose you to weight gain? Is this state your destiny? Can we alter our microbial heritage through our diet, sleep, exercise, and overall lifestyle and environmental interactions? Let's begin with the microbial community itself. In mouse studies, when a large sample of microbiota (organisms of the microbiome) from an overweight mouse was administered into a thin mouse, the thin recipient very quickly began to gain weight. These experiments illustrate that the microbiota can predispose the host to weight gain.

In another study, when comparing stool samples of overweight and normal-weight children, researchers found that there was less bacterial diversity, or less different types of bacteria, in the overweight kids. In an attempt at weight loss, those overweight children with less diverse bacteria had overall less weight loss on the same diet as those with a more diverse microbiome.

Through these studies, we find that microbiome diversity is very important for optimal health. It is no different when it comes to balancing the symptoms of PCOS. But how can this be done? Let's start with what we know can negatively impact our gut bugs:

1. **Smoking**—Smoking causes changes in the mucus profile, diversity of the microbiome complex, and immune factors. Bacteroidetes, with their increased toxins, are increased. Toxic *Clostridium* bacteria are also significantly increased. Healthy Actinobacteria and Firmicutes, as well as *Bifidobacteria* and *Lactobacillus,* are decreased. Suggested mechanisms to explain

the effect of smoking on intestinal microbiome include increased "oxidative stress," which is a chemical process that creates higher numbers of free radicals, weakening of intestinal tight junctions and development of "leaky gut" (where undigested food particles, or even toxins, "leak" out into the bloodstream), as well as disturbance of the acid-base balance. Interestingly, some smoking-induced alterations of intestinal microbiome resemble those demonstrated in conditions such as inflammatory bowel disease and obesity.

2. **Alcohol**—Consumption of alcohol causes an increase in oxidative stress/free radicals, intestinal hypermobility, dysbiotic changes (i.e., the ratio of good bacteria to bad bacteria starts to shift to favor the bad guys), and systemic gut inflammation. While the polyphenols of red wine have been seen in some studies as possibly having some benefit to some species in the microbiome, studies have shown that drinking wine is beneficial to health but only in small amounts (around three drinks per week for women). In a subgroup of people with an alcohol addiction, alcohol consumption is linked with tissue injury and organ dysfunction, increased risk of developing cancer, abnormal function of the immune system that increases the risk of acute and chronic infections, pancreatitis, heart disease, and disruption of the circadian clock. Our 24-hour internal clock, which is one of the most important life forces, can be disrupted by our choice to drink or not to drink. While not judging personal habits, it is important to understand that daily alcohol consumption for 10 weeks altered the colon or large intestine lining and the composition of the bacterial microbiota in rats. It is important to recognize that this disruption of the microbiome composition may be an important mechanism of alcohol-induced endotoxemia. *Endo* means inside, and *toxemia* means harmful substances.

Some of our friendly gut bugs do contain harmful substances in them. When they die, these toxins get released. It is interesting to note that these internal microbe toxins are also released every time we eat. Perhaps that is why intermittent fasting is helpful and has been around for so long. It is a type of gastrointestinal-microbe reset.

How much is too much alcohol? Since alcohol can either be a medicine or a poison, its exact amount for promoting health is unclear, but the general medical consensus today is no more than one drink per day for women. And, yes, having all seven drinks for the week in one day would have a very negative impact on your microbiome!

3. **Chronic stress**—Some conditions linked to stress include irritable bowel syndrome (IBS), food sensitivities, reflux, altered gastrointestinal (GI) motility, and changes in intestinal microbiota. Healthy gut function has been linked to normal central nervous system (CNS) function. The stress response is controlled by the triangle of the hypothalamus, pituitary, and adrenal glands, also known as the HPA axis. Hormones, neurotransmitters, and immunological factors released from the gut are known to send signals to the brain either directly or via autonomic neurons. The existence of the gut-brain axis was proposed in the landmark study by Sudo and colleagues. This groundbreaking research found that the stress response in germ-free (noncolonized microbiome) mice was abnormal. Their stress response was overactivated when the gut microbiome was not present. See Figure 5 for a visual description of the stress response.

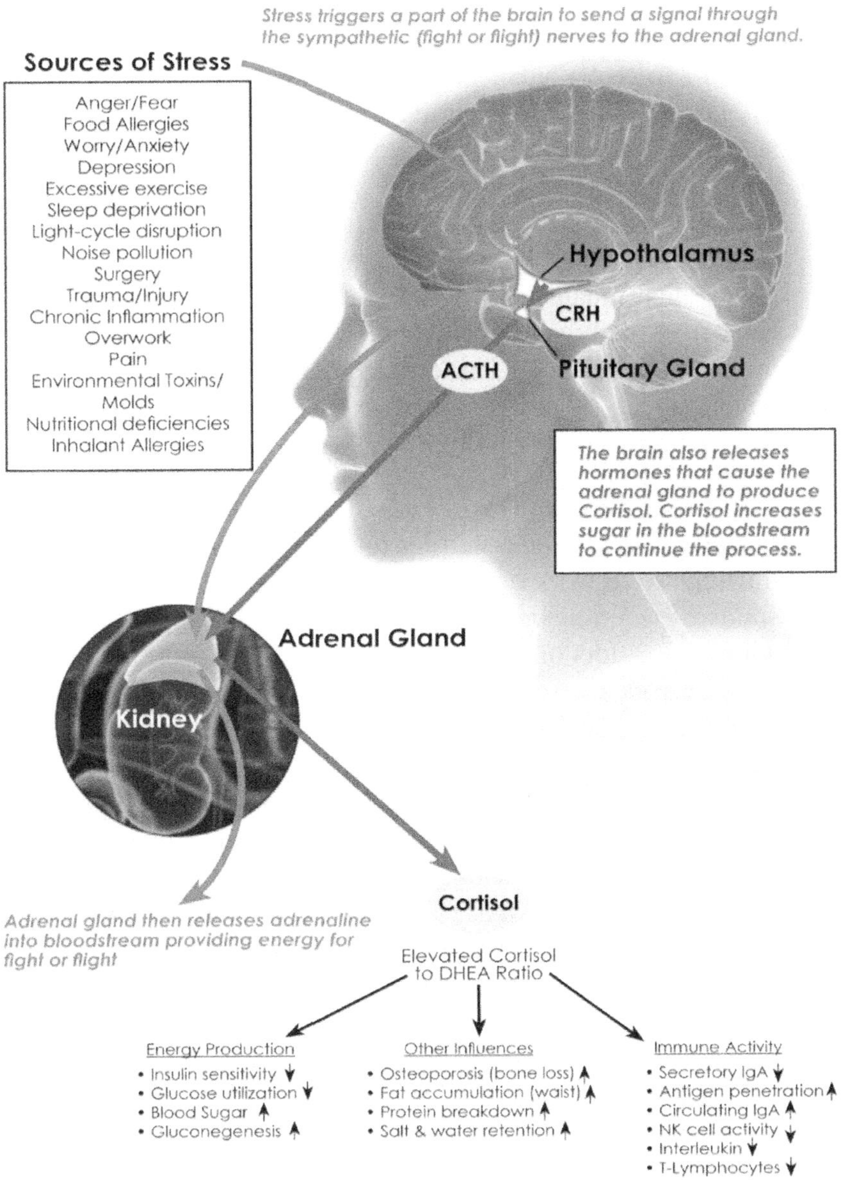

Stress triggers a part of the brain to send a signal through the sympathetic (fight or flight) nerves to the adrenal gland.

Sources of Stress

Anger/Fear
Food Allergies
Worry/Anxiety
Depression
Excessive exercise
Sleep deprivation
Light-cycle disruption
Noise pollution
Surgery
Trauma/Injury
Chronic Inflammation
Overwork
Pain
Environmental Toxins/
Molds
Nutritional deficiencies
Inhalant Allergies

Hypothalamus

CRH

ACTH   **Pituitary Gland**

The brain also releases hormones that cause the adrenal gland to produce Cortisol. Cortisol increases sugar in the bloodstream to continue the process.

Adrenal Gland

Kidney

Adrenal gland then releases adrenaline into bloodstream providing energy for fight or flight

Cortisol

Elevated Cortisol to DHEA Ratio

Energy Production
• Insulin sensitivity ↓
• Glucose utilization ↓
• Blood Sugar ↑
• Gluconegenesis ↑

Other Influences
• Osteoporosis (bone loss) ↑
• Fat accumulation (waist) ↑
• Protein breakdown ↑
• Salt & water retention ↑

Immune Activity
• Secretory IgA ↓
• Antigen penetration ↑
• Circulating IgA ↑
• NK cell activity ↓
• Interleukin ↓
• T-Lymphocytes ↓

Figure 5. Chronic stress response. ACTH stands for adrenocorticotropic hormone, and CRH represents the corticotropin-releasing hormone— these two hormones influence the production of cortisol in the adrenal glands

Short-term exposure to stress within the brain can impact the delicate microbe balance. *Excess* stress will decrease the percent of *Lactobacillus* and dramatically affect the set point for significant anxiety and behavior changes and affect the overall normal functioning of the HPA stress axis. These changes seem to be associated with alterations in microbiota-related metabolites. This means that the waste or byproducts of the "bugs" that inhabit us will affect how we feel. These byproducts can affect the breakdown of important neurotransmitters, leading to brain imbalance. These systems may be important in the development of stress-related conditions including depression and memory loss.

Stress in our modern world is still processed in primitive ways. When you see a tiger starting to chase you (or you are stuck in traffic, have a work deadline approaching, have a fight with your spouse, etc.) you become stressed and need to run. You make adrenaline—lots of it! This hormone is very short acting, and as long as you keep running (or mentally stressing!) you need to keep feeding the adrenaline.

Cortisol is activated as the stress continues to add glucose to the bloodstream for immediate energy and more adrenaline. Measuring cortisol is a great way to evaluate stress and its impact on the HPA axis. The best way to do this is through a four-point salivary cortisol test done throughout the course of a day. *You cannot do a random blood cortisol to evaluate your overall HPA axis as cortisol spikes often throughout the day* (Figure 6). Unfortunately, many physicians will use blood during their testing because that is the standard of care for *disease evaluation* of the adrenal glands. However, this will not tell you the impact that stress is having on your general health.

Once you've determined your cortisol response, use the Roadmap to guide appropriate lifestyle changes. There are supplements that can help with cortisol control, but it's best to use those temporarily as you address the real cause of your chronic stress. Normalizing cortisol will take the pressure off the gut microbiome and let your bugs get back to their "normal life." Remember, they are simply *working with you* in a beneficial relationship. If you take care of them, they will do the same for you. Cortisol is hurtful to them when it is not flowing in an organized fashion at appropriate levels. Test it and fix it if needed.

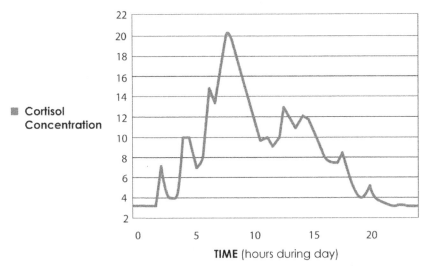

Figure 6. Normal cortisol fluctuations throughout the day

4. **Sugar and processed food**—The gut microbiome is incredibly dynamic and can respond to diet changes very quickly. For millions of years, humans have shared an ever so important relationship with the microbiome that inhabits our GI tract. We fed them seasonally and made sure they had folate from vegetables to make our building blocks of life. Next time you eat, think hard about from what that food is made. Will your gut bugs recognize it as the nourishment they need? Much of the food on our shelves today is more like acid rain to your bugs. It's disguised as something nourishing but destroys them on impact. What is actually in the food we eat today can be detrimental to our own gut and have a huge impact on not only our own health but also the microbiome we pass onto our offspring. It is imperative that you know what is in your food.

In the paper "The Western Diet: Microbiome-Host Interaction and Its Role in Metabolic Disease," Zinocker and colleagues stated the following:

> The most extensively processed foods, termed "ultra-processed," have been defined as "industrial formulations made entirely or mostly from substances extracted from foods (e.g., oils, fats, sugar, starch, and proteins), derived from food constituents (e.g., hydrogenated fats and modified starch), or synthesized in laboratories from food substrates or other organic sources (e.g., flavor enhancers, colors and several food additives used to make the product hyper-palatable).

> To improve food production practices, we propose a new, governmentally directed labeling system, where processed foods are labeled by the level of processing, the addition of additives, and other substitutions for raw material as well as by the percentage of whole foods present in the finished product.

Convenience food may save you some time, but at what price to you and your future offspring?

5. **Antibiotic use**—Antibiotics have arguably the most significant impact on the gut. One Augmentin pill, a popular brand of the antibiotic penicillin, wipes out 90% of your entire microbiome. A 5-day course of oral antibiotics modifies the gut microbiome for up to 4 weeks before it starts to return to normal. When it does return to normal, instead of having an acidic environment, it returns to a more alkaline level, which can promote the growth of the more harmful bacteria. The pH scale runs from acid 1 to alkaline 14, and a healthy stomach environment is acidic and has a very low pH, i.e., very close to 1.

The large intestine, when healthy, has a pH of 5.5–7. The beneficial microbes (flora) that are part of our colon need the lower pH. When the pH is greater than 7, the normal flora cannot live well and the less optimal opportunistic bacteria take over. It would be like trying to live on earth if you woke up one day and the amount of oxygen was significantly lower. You could not breathe, so you could not live. Such is the case here. Eventually the normal pH and flora try to return, but if the wall of the large intestine is damaged and the bad bugs have taken over the neighborhood, then re-establishing normal life is very difficult. You will try to go about your life relying on all the things your normal flora used to perform for you, such as digestion and nutrient absorption, but the good guys are no longer in charge. Many GI symptoms and disease can be explained in this way.

The important takeaway message is that you must be very careful when taking any type of antibiotic. Yes, antibiotics can be lifesaving when an actual bacterial infection is present. But viral infections such as the cold and flu do not respond to antibiotics and can be resolved with rest and nutritional therapies. If you *do* need to take antibiotics, tips to get your gut back on track are included in the Roadmap.

6. **Gluten, glyphosate, and toxins**—These proteins and toxins can cause chronic inflammation that leads to leaky gut and illness, even if you do not have celiac disease. Just like most health fads, going gluten-free has gotten both very positive and negative attention in the press. Celiac disease is the most recognized diagnosis related to gluten ingestion; however, the literature is now recognizing nonceliac gluten sensitivity as a state of dysregulation that can cause not only GI symptoms but also foggy thinking, headaches, joint and muscle pain, fatigue, depression, and dermatitis.

When gluten enters the intestinal lumen or center, it is like a firecracker flowing by a bunch of matches, waiting to be lit. Gluten is a substance present in most genetically modified crops in the US and those heavily sprayed with the weed killer Roundup. The glyphosates in Roundup may not affect your cells directly, which is why the government allows its use; however, it will wreak havoc on your good gut bugs and create the perfect environment for gut dysbiosis or disharmony. Monsanto, the manufacturer of Roundup, just awarded $289 million in damages to a man who developed non-Hodgkin's lymphoma after being found that it intentionally concealed the health risks of its daily used Roundup products. Other toxins in our environment, food, and skincare products can also wipe out some species of our good bacteria and favor other, less friendly, but heartier strains.

Mind Your Microbiome

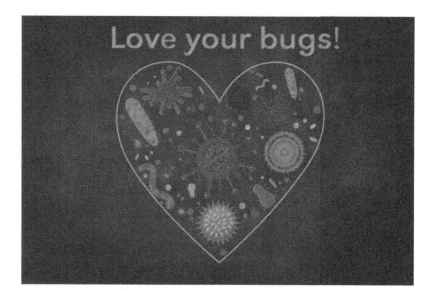

To ensure an optimal internal environment we must nourish it lovingly. One of the best ways to nourish this internal environment is to digest your food well. Our microbes are capable of producing life-giving products for us. The ability of our microbiome to enable us to obtain energy and survive depends on many factors. The two most important are the nutrients we provide with our everyday diet and the state of well-being of the actual lumen or lining of our gut. In a well-balanced state, healthy fermentation of nondigestible carbohydrates (resistant starches) and fibrous vegetables will produce butyrate, an important short-chain fatty acid (SCFA). Visualize this as trillions of microbes jumping on the asparagus or salad leaves you just ate. They then flow through your large intestine, producing products that you can use as building blocks for your GI system and then jump off again. It would be like you, in the right conditions, actually producing the wallpaper that lines your house.

Healthy fat products help maintain optimal colon cellular health while also serving as the basis of much of our energy production system. Each day the large intestine works very hard and sheds millions of cells that are damaged in the digestive process. Healthy levels of SCFA have been shown to prevent or reverse the metabolic syndrome that very often develops as part of PCOS. These SCFAs also minimize inflammatory bowel disorders and keep certain types of cancers from developing.

Many other valuable products are also produced with adequate digestion and bacterial balance. *Bifidobacterium*, as described above, can generate necessary vitamins such as thiamine (B1), riboflavin (B2), biotin, B12, and K2. If you are supplementing with biotin to help your hair and nails, you must consider the state of your gut: What has happened to your *Bifidobacterium* levels that has created a need for biotin supplementation? When our normal bacterial flora is optimized, then pathogens will stay at minimal levels when they pass through our system. Toxins are kept at a low level, and symptoms of bloating, diarrhea, and constipation do not occur. We understand a broken or sprained ankle—having a broken or sprained gut is no different. Figure 7 shows what can happen to the intestinal lining when stress, poor digestion, and toxins overwhelm the body.

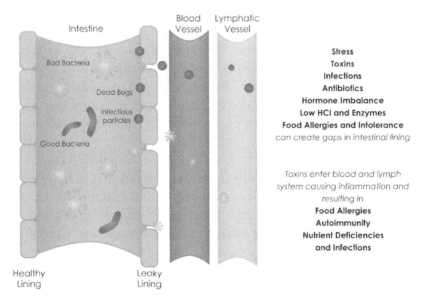

Figure 7. How leaky gut develops

There are no pain fibers inside the intestinal lumen, so we only know something is off in the gut when we experience symptoms such as bloating and gas and/or miserable stool changes. Most physicians only test for a level of overgrowth of bacteria or parasites that is large enough to be considered a disease. If not present, you will be considered normal. However, the absence of disease does not ensure the presence of optimal wellness and optimal balance of the gut microbes. Even a slight shift in the gut microbiome balance can cause constipation, fatigue, and weight loss resistance. One reason for this is poor production of microbial enzymatic activity when the microbiome population is not as diverse as needed.

Digestion is the process that breaks down our food into accessible pieces for our cells and our microbes. The process of digestion should be treated with the utmost respect—faulty digestion starves our bugs and us! If we do not eat a balanced diet for our microbial friends, they will shift to levels that eventually prevent healthy digestion.

For example, a diet too full of simple carbohydrates and not enough healthy fats will eventually lead to poor production of pancreatic lipase. This important enzyme ensures the complex chemical bonds of fat are broken down so the fat molecules can be used for energy. Always remember that we extract more long-lasting energy from a small molecule of fat than the same molecule of glucose. Being constantly hungry or "hangry," especially if sugar cravings are present, is a sign that fat digestion is hindered. The yeast that loves glucose and simple sugars will overgrow and make us crave more and more carbohydrates to feed it. This is common to people who feel they need to eat every 2 hours or they get dizzy.

Animals in the wild are forced to eat a seasonal diet as they scavenge their food every day and may go days without eating. Do you think a tiger ever gets hypoglycemic? It keeps a diverse collection of gut bacteria enabling it to digest whatever it happens to eat. Certain strains of differing microbes will increase in percentage depending on what is available seasonally. A tiger in the wild eats instinctually to feed its microbiome so that these bugs can rely on the slower burning fat molecules when necessary. The Roadmap will help you determine what steps to take to ensure the bugs in your gut are happy and healthy enough to promote proper digestion.

Your Gut Is Your Second Brain

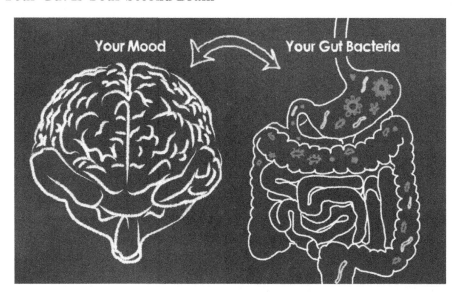

What does your gut have to do with your brain? The microbes in your large intestine are a big part of the neurotransmitter/hormone cascade. The ovaries tend to get all the credit, but a large part of your hormone production and the optimization of its balance happen in your GI system.

The microbiome is actually the master control of hormone balance. The microbes produce and secrete virtually every hormone the body utilizes. All the science and further details that explain this concept can be learned from Dr. Kiran Krishnan in his podcasts. He explains that the microbiome not only regulates the *expression* of the hormones but also inhibits or enhances the *production* of certain hormones, especially estrogen, all over the body.

A healthy microbiome makes, modulates, and consumes estradiol while it produces estriol. Estriol is a weak estrogen that was traditionally thought to be present only in pregnancy. We now understand that it is always present and instrumental in keeping intestinal junctions tight and not leaky. This weak estrogen dissolves easily in our blood to be removed without issues in the liver and helps minimize osteoporosis. It balances the estradiol, which is a more aggressive estrogen, as it passes through a more toxic stage on its way to elimination. The GI tract is also home to the estrobolome—microbes that aid in estrogen elimination. Without an appropriate amount of estrobolome, you will not break down estrogen properly.

We will discuss the reproductive hormones in more detail in a later chapter, but our focus now is that the microbiome produces and secretes 90% of serotonin (the feel-good hormone). This means that the microbiome really controls our mood. Serotonin is also more commonly known as a neurotransmitter, which is a substance that enables information to be passed from one nerve cell to another. Serotonin is the master computer between the gut and the brain, alters mood, modulates sleep, and increases your parasympathetic response so you can rest, digest, and detox. Fat digestion and the breakdown of those more complicated molecules are especially sensitive to loss of serotonin, resulting in too much of an increased sympathetic response (fight or flight). This can also lead to more sugar cravings as the body is not able to extract energy from fats well and is relying solely on the production of glucose from simple carbs. This can result in the following domino cascade:

Excess inflammation → infection → antibiotics → gut dysbiosis → poor digestion → overreliance on energy from glucose metabolism due to poor fat digestion → increased sympathetic response → development of PCOS

The gut also produces dopamine (the motivation hormone/neurotransmitter). If the intestinal system's microbes are unbalanced, then not enough dopamine is produced. Dopamine is the chemical that triggers our happy reward system. A good cup of coffee hits the dopamine receptors and makes you feel ready for the day. We should make enough natural dopamine that the sunshine and flowers and smiles of life give us satisfaction. When the gut is in a state of dysbiosis, dopamine can become chronically low, and the receptors do not get triggered. This can lead to an overall feeling of unrest and apathy. This will drive you to seek external factors to raise dopamine such as processed sugar, alcohol, or drugs. This can be the beginning of depression, isolation, and/or addiction.

Our paleolithic ancestors relied on neurotransmitter balance for survival. norepinephrine (NE), the neurotransmitter of vigilance, kept them awake and alert for times when they had to defend their primitive shelter and food from predators. We still have times today when we need that neurotransmitter to keep us ultra-tuned-in to our surroundings, so NE is still produced to help our system today. Norepinephrine is also produced in our gut by certain strains of bacteria, especially friendly *E. coli*. If there is an imbalance and too many of a certain type of bacteria present, then we will overproduce certain neurotransmitters, keeping us in a perpetual state of fight or flight. This can lead to anxiety, insomnia, and dysfunctional cortisol.

Where Do We Go from Here?

Science is not quite at the point where physicians can do an evaluation of your personal microbiome and mix up the perfect cocktail for you to take as a replacement. I have no doubt, one day soon, you will have a microbiome readout as you breathe on your computer or visit your bathroom that will be complete with your diet and "bug juice" for the day. What we do know now is that everyone can optimize their microbiome by allowing the correct strains to do their job. Reconditioning the gut to favor a big diversity of healthy microbes is of extreme importance. The more different types you have, the better you are.

Microbiome testing and other ways to optimize your intestinal function will be discussed in the Roadmap.

Chapter 6. Epigenetics: Can I *Change* the Expression of My Genes?

"Your genetics load the gun. Your lifestyle pulls the trigger."
Mehmet Oz

It is not possible to point out one single gene responsible for the development of PCOS, but studies suggest there are *multiple* genetic factors that could contribute to this syndrome. Possibilities include genes involved in the insulin pathway, steroidogenesis (making hormones), and those that are involved in the balance of the parasympathetic (rest) and sympathetic (fight or flight) nervous systems. Genes involved in the inflammatory pathways are also very likely involved in the development of PCOS.

We understand that the main thing you want to know about genetics in regards to PCOS is this: Can you change your genetics to avoid developing PCOS? And if you already have PCOS, will your genetics prevent you from reversing it?

You can think of genetics like cards. You can't change the cards you are dealt, but you can change how you play those cards. The winner-take-all jackpot can still be had even if you are dealt less optimal cards. You just have to incorporate different strategies to reach that jackpot. The Roadmap will help you determine which strategy works best for you, but a brief discussion of genetics can help you understand how your genes are not your fate.

All parts of our body are made up of trillions of tiny cells. Each cell contains its own "brain" or nucleus. This nucleus is where the DNA, our genetic code lives. The genetic code determines the basis of who we are, but it is not our destiny. We all have two strands of DNA. One was contributed by our mother and one by our father. Visualize that our DNA looks like a zipper, known as the double helix (Figure 8).

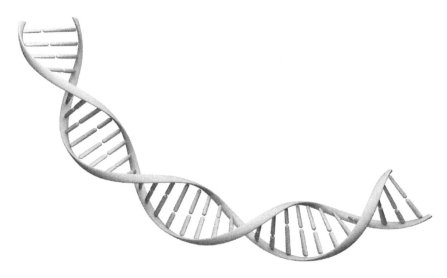

Figure 8. DNA

Proteins that make up all the tissues in our body, brain, lung, heart, and muscle, etc., are constructed based on the orders from our DNA. What is key here is that we can change the orders that are given (the expression of the genes) based on the choices we make throughout our day-to-day life.

The PCOS Roadmap addresses all of the avenues that we can control to determine whether or not the less optimal genes give their particular orders. I use the words *less optimal* rather than *bad* because I do not want anyone to think they have bad genes. Mother Nature is too smart to create bad genes. While we do have some non-needed genes coded in our DNA, nature has carefully devised a mechanism to minimize any of their negative effects. Remember, throughout evolution, we as a race had to exist in times of famine. Many third-world countries still face food insecurity and need the ability to withstand starvation. Genes that predispose to weight gain and insulin resistance to keep life going even with small amounts of food are necessary.

In the United States we do not struggle with famine to that level. While there still exists homeless and hungry people, food abundance is overall our new normal. Winter starvation season for the overall average person never comes. When the hearty ancestral famine genes persist in those that live in abundance, frustrating weight loss resistance will ensue. This is one specific way genes can contribute to PCOS.

The big picture is that we need to turn off the genes we do not need for our current environment. Respecting the light/dark cycle is one way to integrate these ancestral genes into today's flood of light and electricity. We will address this more in the chapter on light. For now, we will explain how the body turns off genes when they are no longer useful. This process is called *methylation.*

A methyl group is simply a molecule made of carbon and hydrogen that comes from the green leafy vegetables that we eat (Figure 9).

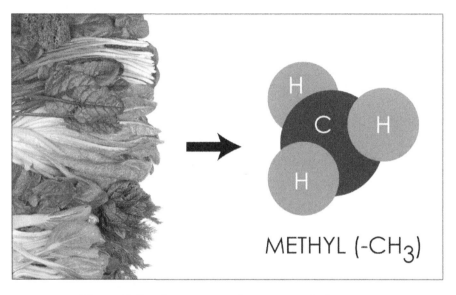

Figure 9. Leafy greens make your methyl groups

We should eat approximately 4–5 cups of vegetables a day for optimal methylation, but the average person barely eats 1–2. Other foods that provide the nutrients for methylation include liver and cold-water fish, which are also often missing from most American diets. In a well-balanced diet, this methyl group is removed and added to B12 to make the molecule SAME. Figure 10 shows all the other factors, vitamins, and nutrients that are important to ensure the cycle spins efficiently. These nutrients must be consumed on a regular basis and are found in whole foods, but rarely in the processed or boxed goods that line the shelves of the grocery store.

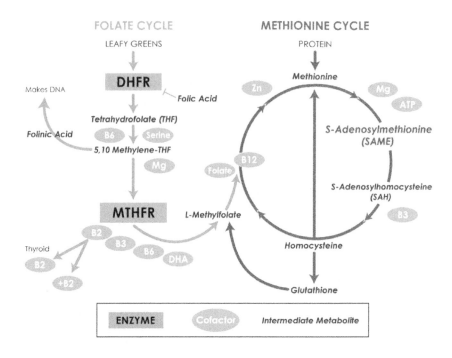

Figure 10. Micronutrients involved in the methylation cycle

SAME then travels all over the body, giving these methyl groups to different cells and reactions. Imagine SAME is holding these groups like a young child holds pegs in the toy Light Brite. Each peg in the toy is a different color. When placed in the right place on a black board, a really cool picture emerges when you plug the toy into the wall and it lights up. So is the case in our body. When each methyl peg is placed in the right place depending on our overall environmental state, the system will run well. Methyl groups can directly affect the development and treatment of PCOS because they do the following:

- Turn off DNA genes we do not want expressed
- Make creatine (the building blocks of muscle)
- Make choline (one of the building blocks of cell membranes)
- Off-load estrogen and other hormones (in Phase 2 detox of the liver; see Figure 12)
- Balance neurotransmitters (controlling mood and premenstrual syndrome or PMS)

How does all of this directly apply to PCOS? The methylation wheel that makes SAME will not turn if the appropriate nutrients are not there, cortisol (our stress hormone) is too high, or our gut microbiome is in a dysregulated state. Eating a typical western diet that is very rich in refined carbohydrates will rob the body of nutrients and often leads to weight gain. When fat cells increase with weight gain, inflammation tends to rise because fat cells secrete inflammatory cells and leptin (another storage hormone to be discussed later). Stress response occurs, and cortisol is released in a constant flow. Your body feels like it is starving *and* running from a tiger all the time, so more sugar is consumed to keep up with cravings. Meanwhile, the gut microbiome becomes overwhelmed with simple glucose sugars, and yeast overgrows. Along with the yeast, the host bacteria ferment the sugars, and the opportunistic bacteria are no longer controlled and hence overgrow. The dysbiotic gut develops, as discussed in Chapter 5 on microbiome, and the culmination of all of the above is that the methylation wheel stops spinning.

The purpose of an enzyme is to help a chemical reaction move to completion efficiently. Our body has millions of chemical reactions going on, all at the same time, every second of every day. The methylation cycle in Figure 10 is one of the most important. If everything in our system is running smoothly, then the wheel in the figure should turn with 100% efficiency. That would be true if all the enzymes were created equal. However, that does not always happen.

Each enzyme is produced from instructions coded by our DNA. When the DNA is assembled, sometimes there occur some changes or mutations or what's called single nucleotide polymorphisms (SNPs). This means, when the DNA was copied from the mother strand, sometimes a wrong piece or base is substituted. So when the code is read to produce the product or enzyme, a little less efficient product is produced. In the case of the enzyme methyl-tetra-hydra-folate reductase or MTHFR (see left side of Figure 10) there are several SNPs that may occur:

- A single **cytosine** is replaced by a **thiamine** at position 677 in the DNA strand. The genetic report would read single or **heterozygous** mutation. The enzyme slows and functions at about 70% efficiency at best.

- A double **cytosine** is replaced by a double **thiamine** at position 677 in the DNA strand. The genetic report would read double or **homozygous** mutation. The enzyme really slows and functions at about 35% efficiency at best.

This is an example of how our body can be affected by our genes in a way we cannot change them. The enzyme cannot work any more efficiently than the DNA has coded it. However, our body is resilient and built to last in extreme stresses, so there is some room for some less efficient reactions as long as the system is not undersupported or pushed over the limit. Your methylation system, even with slower enzymes and mutations, can still perform completely all the jobs it needs to accomplish every day.

However, everything has a limit. The gastrointestinal system is lined with choline produced by methylation. Many processed foods do not dissolve in water and cannot be mixed well with our digestive enzymes. Instead of a cleanly digested mix of nutrients entering the intestinal tract, the package that is delivered from the stomach is full of undigested foreign particles. If contents such as these continuously pass through the intestinal tract, then daily "destruction" will happen to the delicate walls of the gastrointestinal lining comparable to swallowing a firecracker. Not only will the need for choline be excessive, owing to the constant need for repair, but the nutrients to spin the methylation cycle will be in excess demand.

If we are eating many nutrient-poor processed foods and not enough nutrient-dense foods (egg yolks and liver are excellent sources of choline), then the raw material to rebuild the gut lining every day will not be available. Hence, the cycle will slow, and choline will not be produced. The intestinal lining will suffer, and less nutrients will be absorbed as the cells are not healthy enough to do their job. This process will then disrupt the whole system. There will be no SAME for all the other jobs that need to be done such as creatine to make muscle. Your long hours at the gym become a frustrating waste of time as you see no changes in your body composition, menstrual cycle, or fertility hopes.

Here, let's focus on the person who is struggling with low cellular vitamin D even with sun exposure *owing to a genetic issue*. Can supplementing with vitamin D really make a difference?

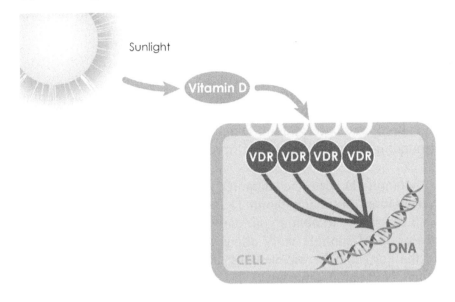

Sunlight

Figure 11. How VDR impacts vitamin D levels

Our body is composed of thousands of cells communicating with each other. The message gets read to the DNA only if it gets inside the cell membrane. Certain gene mutations can make the transporter that sits on the cell membrane move more slowly or less efficiently (Figure 11). Therefore, people with these mutations have less vitamin D in their cells. Should these people live in a place with maximum daily exposure to sunlight, then the amount of vitamin D surrounding their cells all day is so plentiful that the slow movement into the cell is not a big deal. However, should they live where there is rotating cold seasons or work an indoor job, then their vitamin D exposure is restricted. You will have much less D and, coupled with the slow transporter, your cells will feel the depletion. Vital reactions that require vitamin D to occur are hindered. Your body starts to think that you are always hibernating, so it is constantly conserving energy. Hence, your negative symptoms begin. It is now understandable why VDR alterations have been shown to be associated with some of the patterns presented by PCOS.

While studies continue to progress, we do know that within the PCOS realm, the more severe symptoms do correlate with lower levels of vitamin D. Here are some of the more significant mutations and what you should do.

VDR (taq)

The taq mutation in the VDR gene interferes with coding appropriate instructions for making a VDR protein. This receptor allows the body to respond appropriately to vitamin D and interpret the amount of light in its surroundings. Our body can then store or burn energy accordingly.

While vitamin D can be acquired from foods in the diet or supplementation, optimal vitamin D is made from sunlight exposure. That is the best way to obtain your daily dose. Exposing your skin to 15 minutes or so of sunlight daily aligns your circadian rhythm, exposes you to the correct light wavelengths, and creates vitamin D all at the same time. Isn't nature amazing?

However, we must get the vitamin D into the cells. The VDR protein attaches or binds to the active form of vitamin D. This interaction allows VDR to partner with another protein, creating an active combination. The resulting complex then enters the cell and binds to specific genes on our DNA. Turning these genes on or off, the complex helps control calcium and phosphate absorption, insulin use, and overall energy balance. Although the mechanism is not completely understood, the VDR protein is also involved in hair growth.

VDR (bsm)

The bsm mutation is significant not only for receptor issues as explained before but it will also increase your inflammatory load, depending on your diet. Eating healthy foods rich in nutrients without foreign processed particles is very important for health for many reasons. If you have this mutation, decreasing your body's inflammatory load in as many ways as possible becomes a major priority.

Eating organic is a must with this mutation. We are a combination of immune killer cells and immune regulator cells; this balance keeps our microbiome in check. Those that possess the VDR (bsm) mutation have more of a tip to the killer cells, meaning that if and when a foreign substance enters the gastrointestinal tract, more of an inflammatory cascade will occur. Over time this effect will create more negative issues in the gut. Lack of pesticides, toxins, and environmental pollutants in foods are critical in those that possess this mutation. Because probiotics seem to help modulate the immune system, they can also be important for those with this mutation.

The literature is divided on whether having these mutations warrants more vitamin D. I recommend following the basic supplementation guidelines given in the Roadmap and checking your vitamin D levels yearly. If you follow your seasonal circadian rhythms, you will do just fine.

The last part of genetics that is very important to understand is the link to detoxification. No matter how hard we try, we are constantly surrounded by toxic substances that are not beneficial for our body. They are found in the food we eat, the products with which we bathe, and the air we breathe. It wouldn't be optimal for our body to allow these contaminants to circulate through our bloodstream and into the blood vessels in our brain. So, we store them in fat cells. To change a substance that blends with the oil of fat and dissolve it into our water-based blood requires a place and a process. We call that *detoxification,* and we perform that task in our liver (Figure 12).

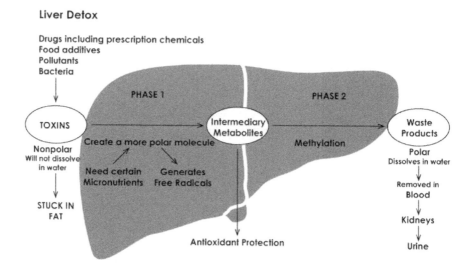

Figure 12. Liver detox phases

Genetically, some of us come from a place millions of years ago that did not require a vigorous detoxification system. Therefore, when there is a strain put on these detoxification cells, they may struggle to keep up. Phase 2 of detox requires methylation, so some women with PCOS inherit a double struggle in this area.

As described in Figure 12, the body can compensate, but toxins in things such as alcohol, processed foods, shampoo, body lotions, simple sugars, and smog (poor air quality) may leave the system overwhelmed. Understanding your genetics just helps you know what you brought to the starting line so you can determine the best path. It is not who you are but what you do with the information that makes you strong.

Chapter 7. The Role of Leptin: Walking the Balance Beam of Life

"Speak softly and carry a big stick; you will go far."
Theodore Roosevelt

We science nerds can imagine that Theodore Roosevelt was referring to the lifesaving hormone leptin in the above quote. Although we don't hear much about this hormone, it controls our powerful central nervous system and, therefore, our actions.

We have mentioned in preceding chapters that the diagnosis and treatment of PCOS have at times been a bit of a "slow-moving machine." One reason is that the largest control comes in one of the smallest packages. It was only discovered in 1994 that a very important master hormone called leptin has a huge impact on brain function, satiety, reproduction, metabolism, fat storage, and weight balance. As we learn more about leptin, we see that it is really running the show. Insulin, progesterone, and estrogen tend to be the main hormones focused on in a PCOS discussion, but to truly understand PCOS, you must know the role leptin plays in the body.

It is helpful, yet again, to go back to the scavenging wild animal model to understand the role of this hormone. In the morning, as the animal wakes after hiding from a predator or sleeping, its blood sugar and fat stores are low. Its body instinctually knows that it needs to move to get food. This is due to the brain secreting a hormone known as ghrelin, the hunger hormone, which sends the body out to find food. Dopamine is also elevated. Dopamine, as mentioned in the previous chapter, is the motivating neurotransmitter that signals that you are ready to take on the world to pursue food. The elevation of these two chemicals in the brain upon waking stimulates the hunting instinct. In humans, the elevation of these neurotransmitters translates to that drive to get up and tackle the world each day. The first bit of food that you eat is turned quickly into glucose to feed the brain.

Once the brain is fed, the body calms down just a bit, but ghrelin is still up. The message is sent to keep looking for calories for the muscles and to store in fat for the future when food is scarce. The body never loses the fear that food may not be available. It doesn't understand the word *supermarket* at a survival level. Robb Wolf explains this well in his book *Wired to Eat*. Our strong survival instincts are always looking to store food for future famine. Our bodies don't understand at a primal level that our current environment has food in abundance.

Once the brain is content, you will continue to eat to nourish the muscles. Muscle strength enables you to build your shelter, run, and survive. However, your body knows you still need to eat a bit more food to save for a "rainy day." Here, you now create fat stores. It is important to remember two very important points: All fats are not the same, and fat is an active substance both receiving and sending out information. It is all about balance developed through cell signaling. Understanding more about the hunger-satiety delicate signaling and where leptin fits into this model is necessary to help follow through on the plan to fix the disruption that occurs. We need to have the right amount of the different fats sending out and receiving messages to keep us burning and storing energy in the perfect ratio. The PCOS Roadmap was created to restore that balance, enabling you to return to optimal health.

Previous research had shown that fat is divided into only two components—white fat and brown fat. But new research has revealed a third type of fat—beige fat. How to maximize the balance among these three fats will be outlined in the Roadmap.

1. **White fat** builds up to develop the pounds we often complain about and wish to shed. But this type of fat performs many vital tasks. Simply, watch an adventure movie where the explorer is stranded in the dark, frozen tundra; it is his white fat that is regulating his temperature and providing insulation. This kind of fat can be subcutaneous (just under our skin) or visceral (wrapped around our vital organs). Subcutaneous fat is found close to the surface of the skin, and visceral fat is found deeper in the abdominal cavity where your precious vital organs reside. Kept in balance, a healthy fat/muscle ratio was life ensuring for our paleo ancestors. In today's calorie/food-rich society,

however, accumulation of white fat that secretes leptin can easily cause us to lose control of the hunger/satiety balance. Once that is in a "free fall," weight loss becomes extremely difficult.

2. **Brown fat** cells contain mitochondria (energy generators), which break down carbohydrate and fatty acids to provide fuel and create heat. Quite unlike white fat, the brown acts more like muscle tissue. *It will actually burn white fat for energy occasionally.* It will also keep you warm when needed by using excess fat stores for fuel. It was previously thought that only babies have brown fat and that it disappears as we enter adulthood. But in 2009, researchers discovered that brown fat does still exist in adults.

3. **Beige fat** has been called "beige" or "brite" because of their intermediate function between brown and white fat cells. A hallmark of these particular types of fat cells is their potential to take on an energy burning role in response to various stimuli such as cold, chemical compounds, or genetic factors. Under baseline conditions, these beige cells express very similar behaviors as classic white fat. They only store energy until appropriately stimulated. At that time, they acquire an ability to increase expression of certain proteins that will aid in increased energy consumption, similar to brown fat.

A deeper understanding as to how and why animals seem to keep their leptin and fat balanced so perfectly will help us understand what is happening in PCOS and how we can address it. What's fascinating about animals in the wild is that they seem to know just *how much* energy to store. Squirrels know how much to eat and store to still be able to climb up a tree and also make it through the scarcity of winter. Birds can eat and store just enough to make it through the flight down south for the winter. Every animal has a certain rhythm with the proper balance of ghrelin and leptin, which tells it just how much food/energy to put into its system.

Once the brain, muscles, and liver are fed and have stored glucose for short-term use (in the form of glycogen), any glucose left over is stored in fat cells for later use when food is scarce. Insulin is the storage hormone that opens up the fat cells to store these nutrients for later use.

Fat cells also secrete inflammatory cells and the hormone leptin. These messages, when read by the brain, will control just the right amount of fat deposition so that the animal never becomes chronically overweight. The following pages will break this down into two parts and address why each is important and what happens when the system gets overloaded.

When fat stores have been filled to the proper level, leptin and inflammation levels have risen to a healthy high. They then send a signal to the part of the brain called the hypothalamus that "I'm full and have enough stored." This signal is received by special receptors on the cell membrane and is interpreted as "stop eating, all is well." The balance of insulin and leptin, along with ghrelin, ensures that the body has just enough to store for a rainy day but not too much so the body can still run, jump, and survive a predator.

Modern life is hectic, and many of us have fallen into a lifestyle that keeps us out of the sunlight, eating convenient, refined foods while sitting most of the day. These convenience foods are super delicious, so it's very easy to eat loads of them. They tend to elevate blood sugar (glucose) very quickly, leading to an almost abnormal elevation in insulin. Visualize this combination like a steam train heading into your central nervous system.

Having elevated blood glucose is very dangerous for the whole body, so insulin has bullied its way into becoming a very powerful hormone. Meaning, even if the fat cells are full, insulin will beat on the cells until they take in the extra glucose.

Leptin, along with inflammation markers, is continually produced by the *white fat cells* with the mission to tell the brain when enough energy has been consumed and we have had enough food. Insulin, however, must also complete its mission to lower blood sugar. Insulin will continue to be secreted by the liver to control the blood sugar situation as long as there is more glucose in the bloodstream than the brain and active muscles need. This is yet another reason why movement and exercise are so important.

While the quality of calories is very important, the quantity of calories does have some bearing. Our body is meant to take in and burn food energy in a perpetual balance. A sedentary lifestyle will lead to a decline in muscle and bone mass. Even at a young age, should insulin see too much glucose in the bloodstream because of low muscle mass and lack of movement, it will bully that sugar into the cells. Inevitably, you will continue to add fat and accumulate white fat cells. And these fat cells will continue to make more and more inflammatory cells and leptin in an attempt to tell the body it's had enough (Figure 13).

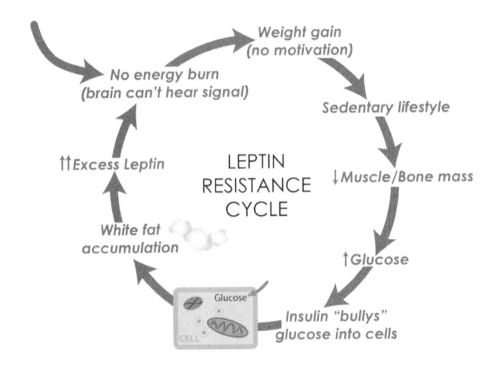

Figure 13. Leptin resistance cycle

These circulating inflammatory cells, along with the leptin, will pulse more and more loudly on the hypothalamus in the brain until the receptors in the hypothalamus cannot hear it anymore. Think of someone calling your name over and over again to get your attention. Eventually you stop listening and tune them out—no difference here. The leptin signal, after pulsing too long on the central nervous system, is no longer transported into the cells. Over time, leptin resistance occurs.

You will learn in Chapter 8 on light that dysregulating your system by not living in sync with the light/dark cycle of the sun will also cause issues at the leptin receptor site. This state is a loss of energy *homeostasis* or balance of use and burn. Visualize confusion when thirty people in a room are all talking about different subjects at the same time with no one listening to each other. Chaos then ensues. In the case of leptin resistance, anything from foggy thinking to weight loss resistance can develop.

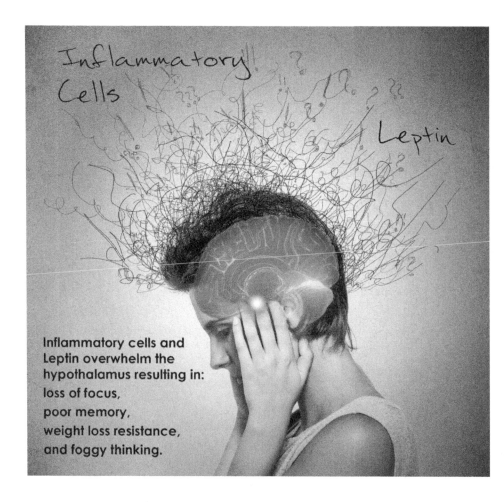

Inflammatory cells and Leptin overwhelm the hypothalamus resulting in: loss of focus, poor memory, weight loss resistance, and foggy thinking.

As discussed previously, fat cells are alive and active and secrete inflammatory cells. These inflammatory cells are a bunch of little particles that circulate around the body, getting into your tissues. Visualize these cytokines or inflammatory cells like leaves flowing down your street in a rainstorm and clogging up the storm drains. The water on the street backs up and can cause problems in the neighborhood. A flood can be incredibly damaging to an entire city, such as when Hurricane Harvey hit our homes in Houston and the surrounding counties. Too many of these cytokines will block the entrance into the brain so leptin cannot enter. This also sets up a state of *leptin resistance*. The fat cells make more leptin to try to communicate the "all full" message to the brain, but because of the increase of inflammation from the fat cells, the signal is jammed.

This is another example of how our bodies have not adapted to the overfed, unseasonal state of our modern world. Insulin and leptin resistance were important survival tools in times of hibernation or food scarcity. These tools are still employed in the animal kingdom. However, the signals of our human bodies seem to be crossed—you feel hungry even when your fat stores are full. This state describes what many patients with PCOS become—a classic "sugar burner." When hunger hits, this woman has a hard time using her stored fat as fuel and must eat again (often craving simple carbs because they raise the blood sugar quickly) to feed the brain and muscles. In fact, a type of panic ensues in the body because the brain needs sugar to survive, but it mistakenly believes the fat stores are empty (therefore, nothing is saved for that rainy day, which is now!). *The body will compensate by decreasing your resting metabolism and actually slowing your everyday calorie burn, leading to increased weight.* In this case, even drastic calorie cutting doesn't work as starvation panic sets in.

This is why it is helpful to know what your blood levels of these markers are. You can look at fasting levels of insulin, leptin, and inflammatory compounds such as C-reactive protein in the blood to give you an idea of the role these guys are playing in your body. Only when the cycle of insulin and leptin resistance is broken can we truly address PCOS successfully. We will discuss this in detail in the Roadmap.

How is PCOS directly affected by leptin and insulin resistance? Each time you eat, you raise your blood sugar. At the ovary, this translates into even higher amounts of insulin floating around. Excess insulin pounds on the ovaries, and more testosterone is secreted. Then multiple cysts develop and PCOS worsens. Even in the system that does not have the myo/chiro-inositol dysfunction, you can see how a PCOS-like picture can develop simply from dysregulated diet, blood sugar fluctuations, and excessive insulin and stress. It is also important to note that making energy out of glucose instead of utilizing fat is less efficient and harder on the body and leads to a greater production of free radicals.

Chapter 8. Let There Be Light

"The eyes are the window to your soul."
William Shakespeare

The eyes are a gift and sight is a rarity when we consider most life forms on earth. The plant kingdom has not been granted the ability to see, and many of the creatures that we interact with every day are using other primitive senses to survive. If we think about evolution, life started under the sea, according to scholars. Of course, there is no concrete agreement on where life began, but most will agree that it was deep in the dark waters.

Scientists look at life on the planet and categorize it into different groups with similar major characteristics or body plans. There are thirty-five different groups or phyla in the animal kingdom, but only six have developed what we know as eyes. What is very interesting is that if we group the percentage of *all* species in the animal kingdom that have eyes, including us, the answer would be about 95%. Clearly, vision was an advantage as the small number of species that did evolve eyes truly dominate animal life today.

Important fact: Eyes develop when exposed to sunlight.

Sunlight, as absorbed by the eyes, was the time clock of life sending signals to the brain to obtain optimal weight, fertility, and survival. The light sensitive cells of the retina are in the back of the eye where they can be protected. Nerve wires guide photons (bursts of light energy) to the correct place in the eye. Right next to the optic nerve is the retina where the received light becomes converted into nerve signals. From the retina, these signals travel into the brain for visual recognition. Blood supply is right behind the retina to bring life-giving oxygen and nutrients to keep the eye healthy.

Interesting fact: The retina consumes more oxygen than the brain for its size and is the most energetic organ in the body with the highest metabolic rate.

The lens that covers the eye is a protein crystal, and the makeup of this crystal is very similar across species. The proteins of the retina are very different and very specialized, but all species have rhodopsin for light sensing. All eyes, from those of the smallest animal at the bottom of the sea with only faint light exposure all the way to our complex eye, use the protein rhodopsin. It is life-altering and key to survival. It is no accident that rhodopsin survived throughout evolution with little change.

The retinal eye pigment is composed of a type of vitamin A. This pigment absorbs a burst of light energy and actually changes its shape. It is usually kinked, but it straightens out with sunshine. And through an open pathway, a cascade of signals is sent to the brain to indicate that it is light outside.

It is the suprachiasmatic nucleus (SCN) in the center of the brain that receives the signal and can adjust what to do with food desires, leptin control, fat burn, and overall energy management. The light lets the brain and our body know what is going on in the external environment. The amount of light integrated by this 24-hour clock regulates our entire existence.

A chronic state of circadian desynchronization may have a harmful impact on overall health and well-being. In other words, when we don't get up with the sun, and stay inside all day staring at computers, we become disconnected to the outdoor light cycle and all the important messages it sends.

Part of what contributes to PCOS can be explained by a lack of light. Remember that evolutionarily, at certain times of the year, insulin resistance, lack of ovulation, and high androgens were necessary to survive through winter and famine. After the long winter starvation time when the body burned the fat stores to live, PCOS reversed itself naturally. Spring came, light filled the sky, and food became more plentiful. Constant outdoor refueling of the precious energy of sunlight spilled all over the eyes of our ancestors, renewed their muscular fitness, rebalanced their hormones, and reignited their brains. Sunlight and its connection to our body rhythms are extremely important.

What happens to blood sugar, fat storage, and hormone balance when the natural sunlight is replaced by the constant indoor lighting and the day and night circadian clocks become disturbed? More importantly, what do we need to do on the Roadmap to return to the optimal state and reverse the developed PCOS?

Before we answer these questions, it's important to understand what *light* really means to us and our survival. At the level of the whole organism, the circadian (day/night) system is organized in a hierarchical manner. There is a master clock within the brain located in the SCN of the hypothalamus. This master clock receives light input from the eye. Nuclei in the brain then transmit timing signals to the peripheral organs on how to do their job on a cyclic basis (Figure 14). This process ensures "phase coherence" within the body, meaning light and dark control food, energy, and general metabolism. In nature today, as animals do not have access to a night light, it still does.

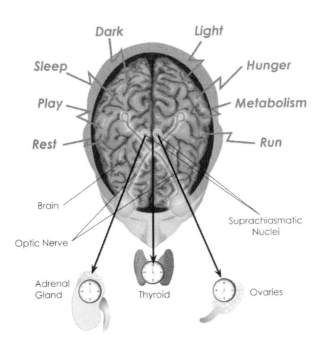

Figure 14. The master clock in our brain

We are living in a rhythmic environment imposed by the rotation of the earth around the sun. Nearly all aspects of our behavior and metabolism are coordinated in a rotating fashion with a period of around 24 hours. It has been this way throughout evolution to ensure the survival of animals and early man. This rhythmicity is set by a group of internal self-sustained *cellular-based pendulums*. Instead of hanging on your wall, the pendulum swings within your body. Of course, you do not have an actual pendulum in you, but your cells have a read on the magnetic pull of the earth and the rising and setting of the sun. This is your circadian clock.

If this perfect cycle is disrupted, the system panics and functions from day to day in chronic stress mode. Every other animal respects the light/dark and environmental cycles on a daily basis. As our brains have developed thought processes and technology that have separated us from our environment, our daily actions are often independent of our light/dark cycle. We have lost key synchronicity in many areas of our body. Realigning with your circadian rhythms and light/dark cycle is a large missing piece that is not often discussed with PCOS healing. But as you now understand, light interacts with your central nervous system, and a perfect balance at the cellular level enables optimal weight, ovulatory cycles, focus, and fertility to occur.

Emerging research has found that direct circadian (light and dark) control of leptin expression in fat cells is just as important as the food balance itself. The response of when to burn fat and when to store it lies more in the light/dark cycle than in the content of the actual meal. That is not to say that if you follow the light/dark cycle, you can pile loads of sugar and refined carbohydrate into your system. That will make anyone sick. What is important to remember is that if you eat a higher amount of starchy carbohydrates in a storage time, you will gain weight, and the clock will not strike for you to lose it, even if those carbs are nutrient dense. Pounding all the leptin and now fat storage molecules into the central nervous system throws off the balanced see-saw (Figure 15).

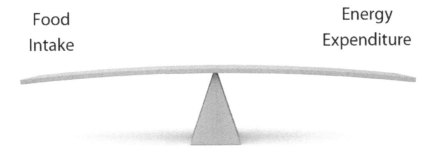

Figure 15. The delicate balance

In our body, there are small molecular clocks in each of our organs. These small clocks not only regulate nutrient uptake, metabolism, and energy storage by targeting the genes controlling the key steps of these processes, but they also respond to changes in food cues and nutrient sensors. The circadian rhythm in mammals is generated by a central clock in the brain that constantly synchronizes to external solar light cues and controls all the other clocks that are active in all of our other tissues. This central clock controls energy use and storage at multiple levels and therefore couples our physical activity, food intake, and energy expenditure with the external 24-hour solar day.

How much we eat and how much we burn are related to the light and dark that cycle around us. Thus, energy balance is a changing and flowing system that is regulated by the light/dark cycle of the sun as seen through our eyes. Loss of this cycle due to lack of sunlight and the current blue lights we sit under all day will disrupt natural rhythms. This eventually leads to underuse or overstorage of energy and therefore excess fat deposits.

Overall, our modern-day lifestyle disrupts different core clock components and causes "chronic social jet lag," inducing similar dysregulation of leptin in the adipose or fat tissue. Distinct body weight issues seem to correlate more with central nervous system (CNS) responses or disruption of responses. Thus, chronic dysregulation of circadian rhythms induces leptin resistance, independent of other known risk factors including gene mutations, diet choices, excess food intake, and sedentary lifestyles.

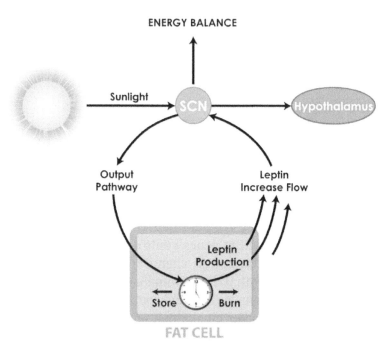

Figure 16. Impact of the sun on leptin

You can buy all the books on insulin resistance and PCOS you can find, but if the central nervous system's light and dark clock is disrupted, the body as a whole stays in a tailspin (Figure 16). Subsequently, the fat is never mobilized to be burned, and the weight keeps increasing. Inflammation comes along and fatigue sets in, leading to less movement. Gut dysbiosis ensues, and neurotransmitters dysregulate as described in Chapter 5 on microbiome.

Studies suggest that although the fat tissue clock drives daily oscillation or fluctuations of leptin, the circadian control of leptin-responsive neurons in the CNS plays a more dominant role in the homeostasis of the leptin-endocrine feedback loop. In plain speak, *light controls leptin, and hence weight loss, more than food does.*

Lack of appropriate vitamin D will further offset this system. Cortisol, melatonin, the main hormones involved in the regulation of sleep/wake cycles and core body temperature, all integrate to enable perfect energy balance (Figure 17). As discussed in Chapter 6 on genetics, let's say you have a mutation in the gene that does not allow vitamin D to easily enter your cells. Should that be compounded with lack of light, your brain and body think it is always winter. This causes cortisol/melatonin pattern disruption.

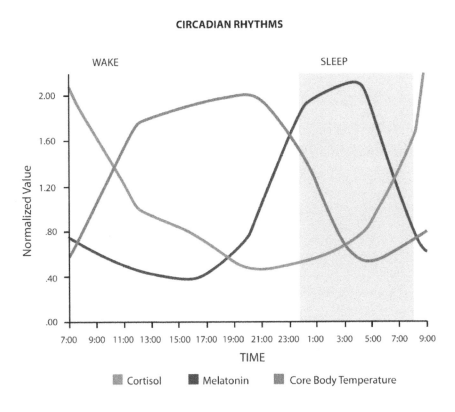

Figure 17. Integration of cortisol and melatonin with body temperature

Vitamin D deficiency has been shown to be a factor in the development of PCOS, and vitamin D supplementation can play a role in preventing this condition. There have been studies suggesting that vitamin D levels are related to body mass index (BMI) in obese patients with PCOS and that vitamin D administration has a positive effect on clinical and biochemical symptoms. However, understand that low vitamin D is not the cause, but the result, of the dysfunction of our present-day environment.

The PCOS Roadmap will help you add light back into your day and guide you through tools that can be added to our sunshine-restricted life.

Chapter 9. Electromagnetic Fields and Their Disruptive Forces

"The pessimist complains about the wind; the optimist expects it to change; the realist adjusts the sails."
William Arthur Ward

Our world revolves around technology. Much of our society is kept in order using computers that regulate sanitation, keep enough food in the grocery store, control traffic lights, and connect us to 911 to save our lives. Each of these devices connects us through an energy highway. So how could something so important and helpful to society affect us in a negative way?

We and the world around us are all composed of particles or atoms. Each atom has a positive and a negative component to it. The positive parts are called *protons* and the negative parts are called *electrons* (Figure 18).

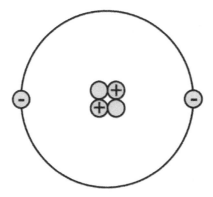

Figure 18. The atom

When the charges are balanced, the forces are all equal, and we call that state *neutral*. When these charges are not in balance because the protons and electrons become separated, energy is created. This energy is then harnessed and used to power our body's functions every day.

While food is often discussed in terms of taste, we really consume our meals to take the electrons from the digested material and give the electrons to our cells. Each individual cell in our body contains a tiny factory. We typically think of workers in a factory assembling or putting pieces together to create a product. For example, all the parts of a car are placed along an assembly line. Each piece is placed, in order, onto the car as it travels down the assembly line. The finished automobile is ready to be shipped to a local dealer and sold for a good price. Imagine the line in reverse. A completed car is placed on the line and each piece is removed and carefully boxed to be sent to different buyers. Someone wants the headlights or the engine, etc. Each piece will bring in its own cash and benefit to the seller. That is how we need to think of our food intake. It is placed on a reverse assembly line where the optimal parts are kept and used while the nonusable trash is discarded or eliminated. Your microbiome, as previously discussed, makes many of these precious decisions. What does all this have to do with electrons, electromagnetic fields (EMFs), and our cell phones? Everything!

A basic definition from the National Institute of Environmental and Health Sciences describes EMFs this way:

> Electric and magnetic fields (EMFs) are invisible areas of energy, often referred to as radiation, that are associated with the use of electrical power and various forms of natural and man-made lighting. EMFs are typically characterized by wavelength or frequency into one of two radioactive categories:
> 1. Non-ionizing: low-level radiation which is generally *perceived* [emphasis added] as harmless to humans
> 2. Ionizing: high-level radiation which has the potential for cellular and DNA damage.

Again, the precious cargo taken from your food is electrons. They are housed in what we call the macronutrients (carbs, fats, and proteins) of our diet. As your food is broken down, the pieces are brought to each of your individual cells to be processed. The cell membrane has a receptor or a door that allows these particles in so the cell may use what it needs to make proteins and energy (see Figure 19 for an explanation of the anatomy of the cell). Your DNA codes for proteins and mitochondria (the cell powerhouses) to make energy for you.

CELL ANATOMY

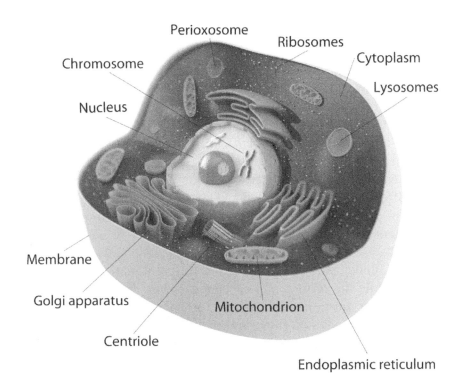

Figure 19. Anatomy of the cell

Without electrons delivered in an organized usable fashion to our cellular components, we do not function well. If the flow of these electrons to and throughout the cell is disrupted, then the cell will struggle to produce efficient energy. The needed proteins or building blocks that are used to keep the brain and the rest of the body running well will not be constructed. You will struggle to make your bones and muscle, as well as feel overall brain fog and chronic fatigue.

Just as cooking and eating a meal produces leftovers, the chemical reactions of our body and the electron flow produce leftover by-products. They are often described as free radicals or ROS (reactive oxygen species). Free radicals are like large taser guns that shock and hurt our cells. In small balanced amounts, they keep our body in check, but in high amounts, our DNA becomes severely damaged and our overall health becomes compromised. How does this happen when using your cell phone and computer? Why include this topic in an understanding of PCOS? Keep reading!

There is something called *non-native EMF* that surrounds us in our technological world and is overwhelming our environment. Your environment is what you are surrounded by every day. Your environment consists of your home (especially your bedroom where a significant amount of time is spent), workplace, and where you spend your free time. In very small doses, this non-native EMF supposedly will not cause harm. However, constant exposure to these waves severely affects our DNA and thus our overall health. Since the body is already in a dysregulated state in PCOS, the non-native EMF bombardment creates a state of further imbalance.

It helps to understand that there are different categories of EMF radiation. While the term *radiation* sounds scary, appropriate doses of native radiation from natural sources of energy such as the sun is actually healthy. Books on the origin of life on earth describe the sun's rays bringing energy to move electrons and current in a favorable way that created the first molecules. These molecules grouping differently over billions of years, along with evolutionary changes, created the organized system (person) you are today.

Your mitochondria, the powerhouses of the cell, have a very similar process that generates your energy, similar to the process used by plants. Plants use sunlight and water in the process of photosynthesis (electrons and current flow as described above) to make their own food. They make much of the food we eat, and their by-product or leftover is the oxygen we need to breathe. We, too, make energy from the sun through skin absorption. Life on earth is basically moving electrical charges that need to be kept flowing and *ordered*. Disorder of electrons in the mitochondria means poor energy production—life then is not sustainable.

It is the radiation outside of these certain natural wavelengths that can hurt us. Waves, in general, have a frequency. Just as the ocean has large waves that roll in slowly and small ripples that pass quickly, so does the invisible flow of radiation passing all around us. Our cells living in a neutral position with balanced positive and negative charges are fine, unless waves of ionizing radiation come pulsing very rapidly into our body. These rapid pulses or frequencies can knock electrons free and create charged particles in us, altering the chemical reactions in our body. While some exposure to ultraviolet (UV) light from the sun is healthy, excess UV on our skin can alter the cell structure and cause skin cancer. If you have ever gotten an X-ray, you know that a small dose is safe, but the technologist who is performing hundreds of tests on different patients wears a lead apron for protection to minimize exposure. We are all familiar with the well-known disaster at the Chernobyl Nuclear Power plant. During the Chernobyl accident, steam-blast effects caused immediate deaths due to a lethal dose of radiation. Over the coming days and weeks, 134 servicemen were hospitalized with acute radiation sickness. Additionally, approximately fourteen radiation-induced cancer deaths among this group of 134 hospitalized survivors followed within the next ten years (1996). Among the wider population, an excess of fifteen childhood thyroid cancer deaths were documented as of 2011. There is no question that this high-frequency type of EMF is a danger.

The gray area regarding EMF danger is the artificial or non-native EMF that technology is flooding our world with today. How did this overpowering evolve? In the 1950s, researchers harnessed microwave radiation to build cordless phones. The problem was that they still needed to be tied to a landline or a base unit. Therefore, your distance from the base was limited to a few feet. On April 3, 1973, the first cell phone call was made. Motorola employee Martin Cooper stood in midtown Manhattan and placed a call to the headquarters of Bell Labs in New Jersey. Ten years later, the cell phone was released to the public. Many say that no product or industry in the history of the world has ever grown as rapidly as the cell phone. Fast forward to today and we find each of our cells and DNA surrounded by smart phones, tablets, and portable computers in addition to television, light bulbs, microwaves, and more. These devices release levels of non-ionizing radiation, meaning the waves do not shake loose electrons to form a charge.

The original research that accompanied these new cell phones said that the EMF released was safe to our cells. Recent studies, however, show that large amounts of these "safe wavelengths" do cause changes in our DNA. As we are electrical beings, these waves affect how our proteins are made and create the baseline of our body strength, the way our DNA is repaired, and the levels of free radicals that are generated.

Mobile phones use electromagnetic radiation in the microwave range (450–3,800 MHz); DNA strands will break when exposed to the 1,800 MHz signal. Other devices that we use daily, including your portable phone, cell phone, cell phone towers, and Wi-Fi router and modem, consistently emit microwave radiation at levels that damage your mitochondria. While they do not produce enough energy to pull the electrons off the neutral particles and create a Chernobyl-type radiation, they do have enough non-native energy to cause the production of free radicals. These waves will produce molecules that are strong enough to remove an electron and damage the DNA inside your mitochondria and the nucleus of your cells, preventing the ever so important organized flow of electrical charge. It would be like putting a big pile of branches across the creek that runs behind the typical country house and feeds its well. Water would simply stop flowing or be greatly reduced, and the family would slowly run out of water. Indirectly, these by-products of the cell phone waves have also been associated with increased levels of systemic inflammation adding to the dysfunction of PCOS.

Earth's electromagnetic field has been protecting all living things since life emerged. Scientists call this the *Schumann resonance* and liken it to the earth's heartbeat. It pulses at approximately 7.83 Hz—a very powerful frequency. In fact, this frequency coincides with the Alpha waves of our brain. This frequency has also been associated with high levels of waves produced with meditation and human growth hormone levels in addition to increased brain blood flow. Our brain can be influenced by the earth's electromagnetic field, which is why being in nature has always been so restorative and healing.

Electron exchange is what makes the world go around. We judge life from a healthy heart (Figure 20) and a healthy functioning brain (Figure 21).

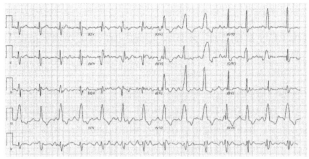

Figure 20. Electrocardiogram

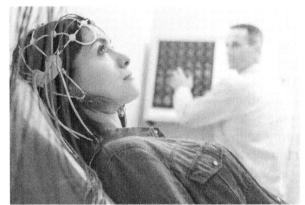

Figure 21. Electroencephalogram

We have already discussed how the brain or central nervous system controls everything in our body. It is like the circuit breaker in the garage. We all know what happens when the circuit breaker malfunctions—the lights go out. This is similar to what can happen in the body: If we dysregulate our electrical current, our system will be in a dysregulated stress mode creating all the symptoms that become exaggerated in PCOS no matter what we eat or how we exercise.

In North America, the power grid we are exposed to every day produces EMFs vibrating at approximately 60 Hz. This frequency alone is way above the natural resonance of the earth and the brain. Existing wires inside the walls of our home and workplace produce EMFs to which we are constantly exposed. Within an ungrounded body (one that has lost direct connection to the earth, as most of us have), electrons and other charged particles react with these environmental EMFs, causing cell and organ function disruption. It does not matter how little or strong the

EMF is; its effect is still felt on the DNA of our body and the computer that is our brain.

One of the most dangerous types of EMF pollution is so-called dirty electricity. This is when the electrical power lines and wiring within your home contain frequencies other than the normal 60-Hz electrical current. These additional frequencies piggyback on the electrical wiring and radiate into your living environment. These frequencies then interact with your body and may lead to the following:

- Headaches
- Insomnia
- Fatigue
- Memory loss
- Heart palpitations
- Mood swings
- Weakening endocrine system
- Poor immune system defense
- Blood sugar dysregulation

We have discussed that poor glucose metabolism and blood sugar dysregulation play a definite part in PCOS. EMFs seem to aggravate glucose transporter genes and increase the production of yeast. Fat digestion in this state becomes more compromised, and the glucose dysregulation worsens. While insulin resistance receives a lot of attention, many women with PCOS do not realize that living in the fight-or-flight state is a large part of what has led them down this pathway.

Emergent research is also revealing that elevated sympathetic (fight or flight) nervous system tone seems to be part of a *genetic component* that predisposes certain women to develop PCOS. Genes regulating serotonin and GABA are altered in these patients with PCOS. While both pathways of fight (norepinephrine) and rest (serotonin) run parallel through the brain, women with PCOS generally have increased norepinephrine levels relative to others for the same stressor. GABA is what puts the brakes on the sympathetic nervous system and calms the body down. GABA is produced by the B islet cells in the pancreas that also regulate insulin secretion. This connection is how your system can decide to relax and store glucose for the future or pour a load of sugar into the blood so your cells can make energy and you can run.

If we follow the pathway, then you can see how the PCOS cycle can develop. With elevated nervous system tone and low GABA, the body is constantly thinking it needs to add glucose to the bloodstream even when you are at rest. If a state of insulin resistance always exists at the muscle level, there is no burn—just constant storage. Not only does this cause weight gain but also all that glucose provides a great place for yeast to overgrow. EMFs will then magnify the damage the yeast can do.

Dietrich Klinghardt, MD, PhD, is a well-known physician who practices integrative medicine. He is focused on the treatment of neurological illness and chronic pain caused by mold toxins. His experiments have shown that mold and yeast will increase their production of toxic load up to 600 times in the presence of EMF radiation.

In the Roadmap, we will discuss how to evaluate and minimize the dirty electricity in your life and help calm your sympathetic nervous system. There is, however, something simple you can do every day to minimize the effects of the EMFs on your delicate system: Practice grounding to off-load the free radicals into the earth (Figure 22).

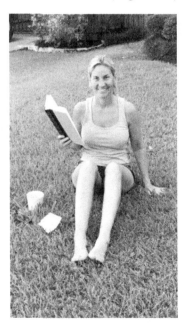

Figure 22. My favorite grounding spot

The land and seas of the earth are alive with an endless and constantly replenished supply of electrons. Since all life in nature makes direct contact with the surface of the planet, our conductive bodies naturally equalize with the earth. Figuratively speaking, we refill the electron level in our tank if it is low, and we off-load the free radicals if they become too high. As the EMFs hit your body from any source, their net effect is cancelled by the electrons within your body supplied by the earth, if you can find some time each day to connect to it. Unfortunately, most of us struggle with this concept because of modern life. However, when we are grounded to the earth, the body is freed of overloaded free radicals and shielded from the DNA disruption by EMFs. Just taking this book outside right now and reading it while sitting on your lawn can be a good first step toward reducing the impact of EMFs on your body.

The main idea of this chapter: Balanced natural energy flow throughout our body is a key determinant of longevity and optimal wellness. Movement and food intake merely supplement and maximize the power field.

Take the time to examine your exposure to artificial light, darkness, and EMF from technology and electric currents where you sleep and live. Tune in to what you do every day, with a new critical eye, in relation to how you make decisions to live your life.

Chapter 10. What Does It Really Mean to Have Balanced Hormones?

"Happiness is not a matter of intensity but of balance, order, rhythm, and harmony."
Thomas Merton

What exactly does *hormone balance* mean? Does it really exist? Those two words are used more often than "I'M OUT!" in the show *Shark Tank*, but often without knowledge of what it really means to be balanced.

Balance usually means stable on each side, which would make us think of a see-saw or a scale. As we know, that is not the case of the normal monthly cycle; that is why we refer to it as a *cycle*. When we think of hormones in PCOS, it would be better to think of a desensitized cycle. By this we mean that the problem lies in the amount of each hormone that is secreted and the absent or poor response of the tissue that the hormone stimulates. You will see in this chapter that different hormones vary in the levels that are secreted each month. We really have to be very careful when we say that estrogen and progesterone are "balanced" in a traditional sense because our body produces different amounts of each of these hormones on different days. It is the amount of hormone produced as well as the appropriate response the body has to each of the hormone surges that are disturbed in PCOS. Thus, we shouldn't make decisions about hormone balance from a single blood evaluation.

Let's take another review of the latest research and how an optimal hormone cycle functions, to help us understand. Then we can approach optimizing the entire hormonal cascade.

Every month, your body wants to have a baby; this is the cycle of life. In the center of the brain is a gland called the pituitary that secretes follicle-stimulating hormone (FSH). The FSH signals your ovary to produce estrogen to prepare the uterus with blood to grow a baby. On day 14, with everything prepared, you will surge your luteinizing hormone (LH) and ovulate. An egg is released to float through your fallopian tubes, hoping to meet a sperm and form a baby. Sounds simple, right? This is the outdated theory of the monthly cycle.

What really happens is this: Our ovaries, pancreas, thyroid, etc., all have their own clock or circadian rhythm and interact with our environmental surroundings, as we've discussed in detail in Chapter 8 on light. Just as animals only reproduce certain months of the year as their reproductive organs interact with nature, optimal food supply, and timing, the early human female was believed to have followed this course. The modern human female in today's society and controlled environment has broken away from the control of nature and can ovulate every month to have a baby. She does this with her ever-powerful brain.

It is commonly believed that the brain stimulates the ovaries to produce estrogen each month in the cycle, but the actual process is much more complicated. Your ovaries, adrenal gland, thyroid, pancreas, and entire endocrine system are controlled by the suprachiasmatic nucleus in your brain. Visualize that the ovaries want to ovulate according to their schedule, but the brain controls the ovarian function much like you control a dog on a leash. It tells the ovary when to release hormones and maintains a very tight control. When the flow of hormones, fatty acids, and glucose and the circadian rhythms are all in sync, we have our monthly cycle (Figure 23).

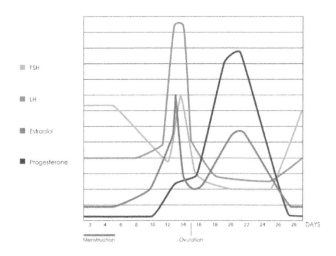

Figure 23. Hormone fluctuations over the monthly cycle

It is the dysregulation of the body's energy flow, insulin, glucose, and light that creates a signaling malfunction to the pituitary gland in the middle of the brain that prevents the organization of the hormone cascade to materialize. Therefore, instead of FSH elevating with estradiol from the ovary and then LH triggering ovulation, the excess testosterone produced in light of the glucose/insulin imbalance causes the wrong ratio of central nervous system hormones to be released. This means testosterone directly stimulates the LH, which rises and creates an upside-down LH/FSH ratio of 3:1—a classic scenario in PCOS.

The result of this imbalance is a steady state of estrogen; hence, ovulation and proper cycling do not occur. This steady state can be low or high levels of estrogen. Estrogen dominance, in the environment of a microbiome that is not optimal, results in the inability to off-load estrogen. The liver's pathway of detoxification becomes overloaded. As explained in a previous chapter, all hormones, including estrogen, are fat soluble as they are made from cholesterol. This means they do not dissolve in water (urine) to be eliminated. They must be processed in the liver and changed into substances that can mix with urine to flow out with our daily waste. This detox process requires two phases, many nutrients, and certain enzymes (Figure 24).

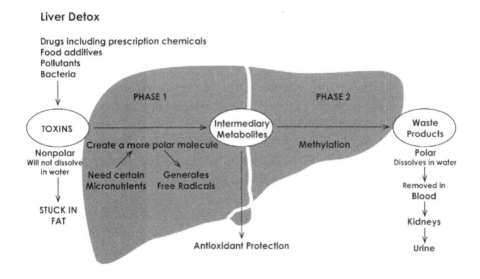

Figure 24. Phases of liver detox

If the detox process does not occur efficiently, the line of hormones to leave the liver will be backed up, and the chronic discomfort symptoms of estrogen dominance such as the following will occur:

- Breast tenderness and/or fibrocystic breasts
- Fat gain, especially around hips and thighs
- Hair loss
- Depression and anxiety
- Mood swings and irritability
- Trouble falling and staying asleep
- Increase in premenstrual syndrome symptoms due to neurotransmitter imbalance
- Endometriosis
- Fibroids
- Low libido
- Water retention and bloating

If you're testing your hormone levels, the most optimal way is through the saliva, not blood. There are two main reasons for this. First, if you look at the hormone cascade in Figure 23, you will see that their fluctuation is so variable that it is only at certain times of the month that any type of ratio of optimization is described. In blood, some of your hormones are free and some are bound to sex hormone binding globulins (SHBGs). Your blood levels, therefore, indicate free and bound hormones, but bound hormones do not affect your deep tissues and your symptoms. Second, all hormones get converted to estrone as they enter the liver. Saliva testing gives you a better evaluation of estrogen dominance by reporting estrone. Addressing low progesterone with progesterone replacement without first ruling out high estrogen issues will be of no help and can actually worsen an already overloaded system. We will go into more detail about saliva testing along with optimal detoxification tips in the Roadmap.

Once you are sure your detoxification system is functioning well and your tissue estrogen levels are addressed, the following are natural ways to help balance your hormones as we are simultaneously correcting all the other environmental factors. Once these and any other dysregulations they cause are modulated, many of your remaining symptoms will be mitigated.

tons of other supplements. The Roadmap will give you detailed tips on improving your digestion.

Micronutrients are the building blocks of healthy hormones; therefore, any deficiencies can have an effect on proper balance. Vitamins B5 and B6 influence steroid hormone production, copper is involved in neurotransmitter synthesis, and iodine and selenium are directly involved in thyroid hormone production. Too much or too little of any of these micronutrients can throw off the delicate hormone cascade. This is why testing can be useful—blindly taking supplements can sometimes do more harm than good.

Follicle-Stimulating Hormone and Luteinizing Hormone

Let's have a look at the FSH/LH ratio one more time. If you do not have normal menstrual cycles and your blood FSH and LH are in a normal range (i.e., not 1:3 FSH/LH but the ideal 3:1), look for other problems that are affecting your ovulation and endocrine system. For example, when blood sugar is dysregulated or when fat digestion is a problem, your cholesterol and whole hormonal cascade may be affected. Very low cholesterol levels (below 160 in some studies) may put undue stress on the liver's ability to produce steroid hormones and seem to increase the risk of anxiety and depression in women. You may or may not have PCOS, but having proper diet and lifestyle to address high levels of blood sugar and SHBG will optimize your body, and your system may normalize more quickly than you think. What I am saying here is that the earlier the dysregulation of the hormones began, the more the electrical system of the central nervous system (CNS) is affected, and the more the FSH/LH ratio will be affected.

Those brain electrical pulses that keep our cycle going is what the FSH/LH ratio reflects. As the ovary of a young girl headed into puberty begins to release hormones, the balance of estrogen and testosterone is very important. When these two hormones pulse at the brain and the testosterone is elevated, the development of the normal FSH/LH pulse is also impaired. Hence, irregular cycles begin from puberty and never normalized. Dysregulation of blood sugar and other effects of the surroundings will affect the "organization" of the hormone cycle leading to this irregularity at a young age. If you are more of someone whose environment created an overall dysregulation after puberty and before menstrual cycle onset, your CNS electrical currents that control your hormone balance were not affected as much. The Roadmap is intended to help wherever you find yourself on the spectrum.

Progesterone Supplementation

Progesterone is the hormone that is often given the most love and respect, so it is helpful to really understand how it is affected in PCOS. It is also often the second thing many physicians reach for after birth control pills when dealing with PCOS. I have found that many functional medicine practitioners are also very quick to prescribe progesterone or some type of herbal progesterone mixture. But my advice is stop, think, address other problems, and see if the system fixes itself before going for hormone replacement. This concept does not apply to the single-dose progesterone withdrawal that OB/GYN physicians often prescribe to clear the heavy uterine lining. But adding more hormones to someone with PCOS who does not feel good, without addressing other issues, is not the answer.

When the brain is successfully communicating with the ovaries and the myo/chiro-inositol balance in the ovaries is ideal, you will see estrogen pulsing with progesterone. However, as already mentioned, the miscommunication that is common in PCOS can lead to irregular and inconsistent release of estrogen, progesterone, and testosterone. With all your other parameters in line, this is where progesterone therapy may be helpful. On day 11, progesterone would start to climb, and then you ovulate. If elevated estradiol is seen in blood, taking progesterone on the second half of your cycle could be very helpful. Since day 1 of your cycle is the first day you bleed, optimal progesterone supplementation should be initiated on day 11 of your cycle. Some choose to start on day 14, but I find better results beginning on day 11 as that is when progesterone actually begins to rise. To follow the natural pattern of progesterone, it should be stopped on day 27 or the first day of menstrual flow.

By mouth is generally the way we use progesterone, but compounding it into a cream is also fine and sometimes tolerated better for certain people. Oral progesterone slows the emptying of your stomach and may cause a little bit of reflux or constipation. Progesterone in cream form may be better in those situations.

A standard dose of oral progesterone is usually between 80 and 150 mg. There is a big difference between bioidentical progesterone and Provera (medroxyprogesterone). Bioidentical hormones are almost identical in structure to the hormones produced by the body, whereas synthetic hormones, like Provera, are structurally different. Provera or medroxyprogesterone is a *progestin,* which means it doesn't fit the hormone receptor for progesterone in quite the same way your own natural progesterone would. It is also harder for your liver to eliminate than progesterone. Bioidentical progesterone will fit the receptor much better and is safe in the long term. Prometrium is actually a bioidentical type of progesterone that the drug companies synthesize. It is safe as long as you are not allergic to peanuts. If you are allergic to peanuts or need a different dosage than 100 or 200 mg (Prometrium or bioidentical progesterone is currently only available in these two dosages), you will need to have the progesterone compounded. The compounded form can be changed to a slow-release version, which is usually a better help with sleep. What I find is that the slow-release compounded products just work better, and I prescribe them as my first choice. Oral progesterone should really be taken at night for best results. It turns into allopregnanolone, which modulates or enhances the actions of GABA, a calming neurotransmitter that helps with sleep. The compounded cream also should be taken in the evening, and rubbing a small part of the dose on the temples of your head can help add that calming presleep affect. The recent studies on progesterone show its safety and health benefits.

Anti-Müllerian Hormone

In discussing hormones and ovulation, I would be remiss if I did not address AMH or anti-Müllerian hormone and its significance. AMH in women is produced exclusively by a particular type of ovarian cells, decreases as we age, and eventually becomes undetectable after menopause. The concentration of this hormone will fluctuate during different phases of the menstrual cycle but only by a small amount. A random sample with accurate results through a blood test can be done at any time.

It is well established that AMH acts as an important inhibitory factor for follicular growth. This means as we start to develop a dominant follicle each month, as described in Chapter 2, the level of AMH elevates and enables the body to calm the follicles, increasing the likelihood of one dominant follicle emerging. This dominant follicle is the one chosen to ovulate. FSH acts in concert with AMH to ensure the perfect balance that is our single ovulation. In addition, AMH has an important role in the ovarian follicular microenvironment. If AMH levels rise too much, this hormone can prevent a single follicle from developing. What develops in the ovary is that string of pearls or multiple small cysts.

What then causes these levels to excessively elevate and how do we fix it? Some have suggested that increased AMH levels result from the excess androgens or male hormones that are produced in PCOS. Impaired production of the dominant follicle leads to accumulation of small, predeveloped follicles. The excess of these follicles may ultimately cause the increased AMH levels associated with PCOS. It is a vicious cycle that feeds on itself. While it seems likely that elevated AMH partly contributes to the anovulation in PCOS, the cause(s) of its increased production to this day remains unknown. The factors that may be involved in the AMH imbalance include increased LH, increased androgen levels, and insulin resistance. Notice that these are the very factors that also seem to be present in most women with PCOS.

What is the actual takeaway message about AMH levels? Ovaries do not function into the menopausal years, and you will see AMH levels drop below 1 in this phase of life. This marker is often used to determine if a woman is in the menopausal stage because it indicates depleted ovarian reserve. With PCOS, however, AMH levels start to climb. In general, an AMH level greater than 3 nmol/mL can be used as a marker for PCOS. However, studies have shown that elevated AMH levels in younger girls can be inconclusive. Following the Roadmap will help minimize all of the surrounding influences on the ovary that create the elevation in AMH, allowing ovulation to occur.

Thyroid

No evaluation of PCOS is complete without addressing thyroid function. The information presented here may be different from what has been presented in the past, but this information comes straight from the latest medical literature. Thyroid information has often been presented incompletely, leading to mass confusion of the general public. However, newest scientific studies are telling us that low normal thyroid is the best thyroid state. This information may be difficult to digest by many because most books on the market blame symptoms of fatigue, weight gain, low libido, poor sleep, no motivation, heavy menses, etc., on a "broken" or low-functioning thyroid. In my office, I have had women break down in tears when told their thyroid levels are normal and healthy or need to be on the lower side and do not explain why they feel bad. It would be such a great, easy fix if simply adding a bit of thyroid hormone cured all these complaints.

The wild is a difficult place to live. We know that transient fasting benefits our cells and mitochondria. We discuss how 12–16 hours of fasting can help us in our modern-day life maximize our longevity. A little stress in any situation is healthy and motivating. However, prolonged and excessive cold and starvation can be deadly. Your body would need to slow down your metabolism to conserve energy on a regular basis. The popular reality television show *Survivor* showcases this quite clearly.

Let's illustrate what constitutes healthy thyroid hormone levels. While some women with PCOS truly have a low-functioning thyroid, or true hypothyroid dysfunction, more often than not, what actually accompanies PCOS is something called *nonthyroid illness syndrome* (NTIS). In this state of function, it is the *conversion* and *balance* of each of the particular thyroid hormones that is the problem. Altered action on your body tissues are the real culprits of the thyroid confusion. The explanation below will clarify how the imbalance previously described is creating what *appears* to be a low-thyroid issue. After reading and understanding where your body has deviated from a balanced state, you will be able go back to the Roadmap and realign your system. Often, without medication, your thyroid hormone levels will normalize.

Alterations in the thyroid hormone economy or balance and production of the different thyroid hormones are the basis of NTIS. Before we discuss the imbalance of these hormones, a brief review of the thyroid is helpful. The thyroid gland is located in the middle of the neck and sits on the windpipe. Producing the hormones illustrated below, they are chemical messengers that suggest to the cell and DNA what is the best course of action for the whole body's metabolism in a particular situation. While much of the basic hormone production (free thyroxine or T4) occurs in the neck gland, most of the conversion into usable products of the hormone happens in the liver. Conversion also takes place in cells of the heart, muscle, gut, and nerves. Jim Paoletti, the former director of education at ZRT Laboratories, described this concept in terms of the thyroid hormone gradient (Figure25).

Thyroid Level Gradient Example

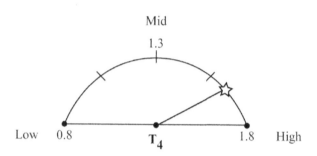

Figure 25. Jim Paoletti's thyroid gradient illustration

We typically think of thyroid stimulating hormone (TSH) as activating the thyroid to produce T4. Once produced, it will be released into the bloodstream to be converted to T3, reverse T3 (RT3), and even reverse T2 (RT2) in the tissues. T3 will send a call to action to each cell to increase its energy/glucose or fat burn. Reverse T3, however, cannot enter the cell; it sits on the receptor and blocks the other hormones from entering. The "turn it up" message then cannot be communicated.

The main feature of NTIS is a fall in T3 levels, due to the overall state of the body, with a normal TSH. A low production of T3 does not automatically mean a poor-functioning thyroid, yet some turn to thyroid medication immediately. Again, fix the underlying problem, look at all lanes of the Roadmap, and see if the thyroid levels are reflecting sickness as opposed to low function.

Remember, T4 and RT3 levels will vary according to the body's underlying dysregulation or illness. It has been known for many years that profound changes in thyroid hormone metabolism occur when one develops sick euthyroid syndrome or low-T3 syndrome. This condition is characterized by decreased T3 and, in severe illness, decreased T4 and increased RT3. TSH is usually normal but may be slightly increased or even decreased. In patients with life-threatening infections, peripheral tissues need to sacrifice to save the brain, heart, and kidneys. Muscle then decreases thyroid production and increases degradation while adipose/fat decreases uptake of T3. All peripheral tissues decrease thyroid hormone actions. The patient is not hypothyroid; the body is merely making decisions to lower the active thyroid hormones, and therefore metabolism, when it is not in its optimal state.

NTIS can be seen as a useful adaptation of the body to counteract an excessive breakdown that occurs during illness. It is part of the acute phase response, which is one of the major defense mechanisms of the body that is predominantly stimulated by inflammation. Remember that the body sees stress and inflammation as all the same. A dysregulated blood sugar system and an altered state of the microbiome are interpreted by the body to be no different than if you were being chased by a tiger. These thyroid abnormalities represent imbalances in thyroid hormone production, metabolism, conversion, and action on the tissues of the body. We must think of PCOS as the body in a stress state due to the insulin, blood glucose, and hormone imbalance state of being leading to NTIS.

Understanding thyroid conversion is necessary in order to know how the imbalance occurs and more importantly how we can use the Roadmap to fix it. The metabolism of thyroid hormones is determined by the action of three enzymes: D1, D2, and D3. These enzymes help the interconversion of T4, T3, RT3, and eventually to RT2 (completely inactive). When the system is not full of stress and inflammation, the enzymes perform their functions and receive the messages appropriately.

Deiodinases (Enzymes that Remove Iodine)

D1: located in the cell membrane and is able to remove iodine from T4. D1 is expressed in the liver, kidney, thyroid, and pituitary.

D2: located inside the cell and removes iodine from T4 to create the biologically active T4. It is negatively regulated by T3. As the amount of T3 increases, D2 expression decreases. Higher levels of T4 and RT3 increase D2 activity; when circulating T4 levels decrease, the enzyme will slow.

D3: also located on the cell membrane and can be viewed as the major thyroid hormone-inactivating enzyme. It removes iodine from the rings of T4 and T3, producing the inactive RT3 and RT2.

Deiodinases are regulated by circulating levels of thyroid hormone. In particular, D2 activity is increased when circulating T4 levels are decreased, and vice versa. Studies in patients with illness and inflammation have shown decreased activity of D1 in the liver and skeletal muscles, increased D2 activity in skeletal muscles, and an increase in D3. This state causes T4 to be converted to reverse T3 instead of the active hormone T3. Hence, we see the classic pattern of low T3 and increased RT3. The enzymes and conversions are on an inflammation see-saw, which causes levels of blood T4 to vary. Therefore, you can have a completely normal-functioning thyroid, but the body creates a dysfunctional pattern based on the state of all its other parameters. Simply adding more thyroid through a medication or supplement is not the answer!

What happens in the case of PCOS? Blood sugar dysregulation, insulin resistance, microbiome dysbiosis, and environmental disconnect create the perfect storm for NTIS. In rodents, exposure to a bacterial toxin showed an increase in D2 enzyme activity in the brain. This illustrates that development of intestinal inflammation and leaky gut will affect the brain and therefore the thyroid. We know that many of these parameters are present in PCOS. Again, it is not about the ever-changing prescription of your thyroid medication, but the imbalance of the whole body. Address the microbiome and decrease your brain inflammation, and you will then begin to rebalance the conversion of your T4 to T3.

As this chapter closes, we must again revisit the hormone leptin and its brain-thyroid interaction. It has been shown in animals that when they are excessively deprived of food, D2 activity is elevated in the brain. This is not what is seen with intermittent fasting but *severe, long-term* calorie restriction. During this food deprivation, circulating levels of the adrenal stress hormone rise while levels of adipose tissue-derived leptin fall. We would expect this D2 increase to coincide with a decrease in the plasma levels of T4 and in an increase in T3 because of the stress situation. In other words, we would expect the body to make more T3 in times of stress to increase the metabolic rate until the stressor is gone. That, however, does not happen. In these studies, when the animals were severely deprived of food, both free T4 and free T3 (*free* means unbound to other proteins and thus more available to tissues) were decreased. Similar to a woman starting thyroid medication, when T4 was replaced in these fasted animals, D2 activity levels were not restored to lower levels. The system was not restored when medication was given, suggesting that *a signal other than that from just the thyroid* is responsible for the regulation of D2 and overall conversion of thyroid levels throughout the body.

Leptin is an important factor in this regard because its levels fall in concert with weight loss. Leptin was shown to stimulate TSH levels, and this finding may help to explain the increased TSH levels often found in obese individuals. Patients who have a defective leptin receptor or leptin resistance show decreased TSH secretion. It appears that in humans, certain levels of leptin are necessary for adequate pituitary/thyroid function. As long as the signaling continues to be recognized between the brain and the leptin, all is good. During severe food deprivation, both T4 and T3 levels are decreased, hence conserving all energy. Under this metabolic condition, brain D2 activity is elevated. *Systemic T4 administration does not reverse these brain changes.* It appears that leptin and cortisol play a role in these mechanisms, and their interactions are an important regulator of the hypothalamic-pituitary-thyroid axis.

Finally, as described in Chapter 7 on leptin, if the brain does not recognize the leptin signal and leptin resistance has developed, it will assume that the body is constantly starving and will signal the D2 enzyme and peripheral tissues to stop all conversion to active T3 hormones. Metabolism and energy burn will stop, calories will continue to be stored, and weight and other symptoms will not change. You cannot supplement and push past what the brain has dictated!

Where does this leave us when it comes to thyroid? I am not suggesting that anyone discontinue their medication. However, I do think that when patients have dysregulation anywhere in the body or environment as described in previous chapters, many doctors (and patients!) assume that levels of T3 and T4 should be closer to the higher side. Actually, studies in 10,000 patients show that higher levels of total T4 and FT4 were correlated with increased heart attack risk. Please do not first reach for thyroid medication, especially if you fall into the normal range, before addressing and correcting the other parts of the Roadmap.

Chapter 11. Recovery: The PCOS Environmental Roadmap

The PCOS Roadmap is divided into six parallel lanes that can and need to be traveled simultaneously:

Each section of the Roadmap is divided into three sections:

DRAW—recommended testing

DO—what you can do immediately to start healing

TAKE—supplements that can be helpful in the healing process. Remember, these are meant to *supplement* the action steps. They should not take the place of the diet and lifestyle recommendations in the **DO** sections. Not all supplements recommended will be needed by every reader.

1) Energy Balance - *Intake and Burn*

 DRAW

Leptin
Levels below 25 ng/mL are considered ideal.

Fasting Glucose and Insulin
The ideal level for fasting insulin is around 7 µIU/mL, and ideal levels for fasting glucose are 80–85 mg/dL.

Ideally, a glucose/insulin challenge test should also be done because a fasting level will tell you what your levels are after an 8–12 hour fast, but knowing how your glucose and insulin react after eating carbohydrate-rich foods is also important. The example below uses a sweet potato to test this, but you could use any carb-rich food that is equal to 50 g of carbs such as beans, white potato, or rice. If you are currently eating flour-based grains, it is a good idea to test your body's reactions to those foods, so choosing something like an English muffin or bagel would give you useful information. The instructions for this test are included below; you will need to find a practitioner that will draw these labs:

Cook one medium sweet potato and bring with you to the lab. You will need approximately 1 ¾ cups. Do not put anything on the potato. Have one blood draw before eating anything, then eat the sweet potato. Wait 1 hour and draw blood again, wait 1 hour more, then draw blood again. Peak insulin should occur at the 1-hour mark, and the second-hour insulin should be less than 50 mg/dL. The second-hour glucose should be between 90 and 115 mg/dL.

If glucose and insulin levels are higher than what is indicated above, that food is causing an abnormal response and should be reduced or eliminated from the diet. High numbers also indicate that the body's ability to handle dense carbs is compromised.

High Sensitivity C-Reactive Protein
The ideal level is below 1 mg/L, but the normal level is anything under 3.

Adiponectin
The normal range is 5.5–37 μg/mL. Values on the low side of the range can indicate a loss of sensitivity.

Functional Testing
The above tests (with the exception of the glucose/insulin challenge) are pretty standard to most physicians' offices and are likely to be covered by insurance. In each section of the Roadmap, we will also cover testing that is more functional in nature. In other words, this testing uses technology and parameters that allow the practitioner and patient to individualize protocols for ideal health, not just disease. These tests are unlikely to be covered by insurance, but they can be particularly helpful in determining the state of your blood sugar and nutrient status.

SpectraCell Labs

- **Micronutrient Test (MNT):** This meas⸱
of thirty-five nutritional components inc⸱
antioxidants, minerals, and amino acids ⸱
blood cells. This test is a great way to determine which
micronutrients are missing and the best way to replenish
them.

- **Cardiometabolic Panel**: This measures fasting insulin,
glucose, leptin, adiponectin, along with a full omega
check and cholesterol panel. This is the test we order
most often on our patients with PCOS.

 DO

Tips to Increase Brown Fat for Maximizing Metabolism

1. **Balance your calories**. This is the Goldilocks rule of healthy
eating—your caloric intake should be "just right." This means you
do not overeat, nor do you starve yourself (which is different from
intermittent fasting). Chronically undereating has detrimental effects
on your metabolism. Body composition testing can help you
determine your lean body mass, which is the best way to determine
your optimal caloric balance.

2. **Exercise increases brown fat**. As you become fit, your brown
fat will increase. Find something you like to do (walking, hiking,
weight lifting, swimming, etc.) and commit to it three to four times a
week. If you are pressed for time, there are a ton of interval
workouts that take less than 10 minutes available on the Internet.
Doing a 10-minute workout twice per day will reap the same
benefits as doing a consistent session of 20 minutes. We also
demonstrate short workouts that can be done at home on our
YouTube channel: dianginsbergMD.

3. **Practice cold thermogenesis**. Cooler temperatures will activate the brown fat in your body and allow you to burn more calories. Consider taking a cold shower or ice bath, turning the thermostat down a few degrees in your home, or spending time outside in cold weather. Exercising outside in the cold weather is a double bonus!

4. **Increase melatonin**. This may be one of the reasons why good sleep helps with weight management since melatonin is naturally at its highest levels in the body when asleep at night. Sleeping in a cold, dark room increases melatonin even more as does consuming mustard, Goji berries, almonds, sunflower seeds, cardamom, fennel, coriander, and cherries.

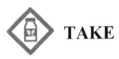 **TAKE**

You want to consume your supplements from a *pharmaceutical grade* vitamin company. All supplements are definitely not the same. Supplements are categorized as nutritional grade, medical grade, or pharmaceutical grade.

Nutritional Grade
Vitamins you find at your local store (GNC, Vitamin Shoppe, Central Market, and Whole Foods). There is no real regulation on these, so you may not be getting the 1,000 mg of vitamin C that they claim. The purity is questionable, and the actual vitamin is in a form that is not very bioavailable, that is, they are not readily assimilated into gastrointestinal (GI) tissues. Some of these brands may contain preservatives, colorings, synthetic chemicals, and other problem ingredients. You have to go above and beyond to find good-quality nutritional supplements as quality standards vary between stores.

Medical Grade
Their bioavailability is better than that of nutritional grade and in a purer form. These preformulated supplements will target a specific function of the body; however, no outside source has evaluated the product and validated its contents.

Pharmaceutical Grade

The best vitamin you can buy. This category of vitamins is formulated with the highest standard of quality to provide the greatest efficacy and quality. For a company to have this claim, an outside accredited lab has evaluated the supplement and confirmed that they are the purest and most bioavailable. Brand-name examples of this class of vitamin: Designs for Health, Orthomolecular, Apex, Xymogen, Microbiome Labs, and Biotics.

1. Omega-3 Fish Oil

Omega-3 fatty acids have multiple positive effects on PCOS as described in multiple chapters of this book. Getting a good-quality omega-3 supplement with the right amounts of this fatty acid is easier said than done, though.

Omega-3 fats are polyunsaturated fats known as essential fats, meaning your body can't make them from other fats; they must be included in the diet. There are three main omega-3s: EPA, DHA, and ALA.

> **Eicosapentaenoic acid (EPA)** and **docosahexaenoic acid (DHA)** come mainly from fish.

> **Alpha-linolenic acid (ALA)** are the most common omega-3 fatty acid found in nuts (especially walnuts), flaxseed and flaxseed oil, leafy vegetables, and especially in the meat of grass-fed animals. The human body generally uses ALA for energy, but most importantly, for conversion into EPA and DHA. As we cannot synthesize ALA, we must consume it. Plants such as algae and flaxseed do contain omega-3s in the form of ALA, but these plants are not converted to DHA and EPA as easily as animal fats.

Quality omega-3 supplements will contain around 500 mg of EPA and 400 to 500 mg of DHA per serving. Some omega supplements will include omega-6s as well, which the standard American diet already contains an abundance of. Also be aware that the source of the fish is very important owing to contamination and mercury risks. Our favorite fish oil brands include Ortho Molecular and Designs for Health.

2. Berberine

Berberine is the active component of the medicinal plant *Rhizoma coptidis*. Chinese medicine has long used berberine for its antidiabetic effects, lipid metabolism upregulation, and improvement of metabolic syndrome. Its mechanism seems to work through the downregulation of the expression of genes involved in lipogenesis and upregulation in those involved in energy expenditure. Both adipose and muscle tissue are positively affected.

Berberine treatment appears to increase AMP-activated protein kinase (AMPK) activity and increases GLUT4 translocation. The effect berberine has on this pathway leads to reduced energy storage and increased energy production. Insulin resistance is minimized, and fat burn is increased. A daily dose of 400 mg is recommended.

3. Diaxinol
This blend of synergistic ingredients by Ortho Molecular aids in controlling blood glucose swings. While lab results may show a certain blood glucose number at a certain time, patients with PCOS seem to have a wider variation of their blood sugar throughout the day and during their meals. With a predisposition to insulin resistance, minimizing those variations will lead to less cortisol dysfunction and fat storage.

4. Metabolic Synergy
This Designs for Health blend is the mother of all vitamins for blood sugar regulation. However, it can be overwhelming to take as the prescribed dosage is six capsules per day. Taking two capsules at each meal will help it absorb better and make it more manageable.

5. Myo/Chiro-Inositol Balance
As explained previously, it is the balance of the two as determined by the epimerase enzyme and surrounding blood glucose and insulin levels that determine how the reproductive system is affected. The optimal ratio is 40:1, so please make sure that the supplement you take contains that ratio. Our favorite is Sensitol by Designs for Health; the prescribed dosage is two capsules, twice daily.

DRAW

MTHFR
C677T and A1298C are the most well-studied types of MTHFR mutation. The mutations with the most significant impact on health seem to be the homozygous A1298C (C1298C), homozygous C677T (T677T), and compound heterozygous A1298C + C677T

VDR (bsm)
This mutation is thought to cause an inappropriate and continuing inflammatory response to foreign foods and microbes.

VDR (taq)
Codes for the vitamin D receptor that enables its entry into the cell.

CYP 1a1
Codes for the enzyme that facilitates the metabolism of estrone in the liver in the detox process.

Homocysteine
Increased or significantly decreased levels of homocysteine can indicate poor methylation status. The ideal level is around 7.

COMT
Metabolizes dopamine and estrogen. Mutations in this enzyme can either speed up this metabolism or slow it down.

Micronutrient Testing
This test helps you determine if you actually need extra methyl folate or other vitamins involved in methylation. Many patients start to blindly take high doses of methyl folate when they discover they have the MTHFR mutation only to find that it leads to increased anxiety. Having this mutation doesn't automatically mean you are low in folate. Testing can help you determine the supplements that are actually needed by the body.

 DO

bel on your supplements very carefully and avoid
that contain folic acid. Folic acid is a synthetic form
tamin folate and can inhibit the body's ability to
al folate. This is especially an issue if you have a
.... this enzyme as your body's ability to utilize folate is
already slower than of people who do not have this mutation.

2. **Avoid all white processed foods** such as flours, breads, rice, and cereal as these are likely enriched with folic acid. Also read labels on energy and protein bars, vitamin waters, and workout drinks as they may also be "enriched" with folic acid.

3. **Take more natural, whole foods** as these are the best source of methylation nutrients: Dark leafy greens are one of the best sources of folate; fish, meat, and eggs provide natural sources of B2, B12, and methionine; nonstarchy veggies and whole grains provide B6; and liver provides all of the above.

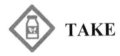 **TAKE**

1. Eat a wide variety of foods, including vegetables (especially dark green leafy vegetables), fruits, nuts, beans, peas, seafood, eggs, meat, and poultry. Spinach, liver, asparagus, and brussels sprouts are among the foods with the highest folate levels.

2. Supplements that contain vitamins D3 with K2 seem to be better absorbed than supplements with D3 alone. Pharmaceutical grade vitamin D will generally have K2 combined in the formula. Optimal vitamin D levels in your blood should hover between 60 and 80 ng/mL. If your personal labs show levels less than this, you can generally raise your vitamin D by 10 ng for every 1,000 IU you consume. International units (IU) currently describe how vitamin D is supplied, although many companies are slowly switching this to micrograms (mcg). It is helpful to work with a practitioner to determine your optimal supplemental dosage based on testing once or twice per year. However, a good general protocol is below:

- On days you have no sun exposure, take 4,000 IU.
- If you are exposed to small amounts of sunlight (less tha
  15 minutes), take 2,000 IU.
- If you have a good day of natural sunlight, take none.

3. Make sure your skin care and hair products are free of harmful toxins and hormone mimickers. Sluggish detox is often a side effect of many of the genetic mutations discussed above, especially MTHFR, so it is important that you evaluate your daily cleansing, makeup, and hair products. Beauty Counter has done an excellent job of outlining what you should never put on your skin as it is toxic to your body (see a complete list and explanation at https://www.beautycounter.com/the-never-list). Here are some of the ingredients to avoid:

- Benzalkonium chloride
- Butylatedhydroxy anisole and butylated hydroxytoluene
- Coal tar hair dyes and other coal tar ingredients
- Ethylenediaminetetraacetic acid (EDTA)
- Ethanolamines (MEA/DEA/TEA)
- Formaldehyde
- Hydroquinone
- Methylisothiazolinone and methylchloroisothiazolinone
- Oxybenzone
- Parabens (methyl-, isobutyl-, propyl-, etc.)
- Polyethylene glycol (PEG compounds)
- Retinyl palmitate and retinol (vitamin A)
- Sodium lauryl sulfate and sodium laureth sulfate (SLS and SLES)
- Synthetic flavor or fragrance or parfum
- Toluene
- Triclosan and triclocarban

Diagnostic Solutions GI Map
This is a comprehensive stool analysis utilizing DNA technology. This test shows the balance of the microbiome along with overall digestive function, inflammation, and immune markers. You do not have to fast or prep for it; you simply send in a stool sample and it is analyzed. Discussing this test with a qualified practitioner can help you determine if any bacterial or viral pathogens need to be removed, the extent of repair needed in the gut, and what microbes need to be replaced.

Liver Function Tests
Liver enzymes such as AST/ALT/GGT levels may elevate when a virus is present. These levels should be monitored until they normalize. Slight elevations are often negated by doctors, but low-level elevation can mean microbiome issues. If liver and intestinal functions are flowing well, there is no reason for the enzymes to elevate. Think of a rainstorm; if the rain is not too constant and heavy and the ground can handle the absorption of the water, there is no flooding. But if the downpour is constant and unrelenting on an already saturated ground, flooding develops. Our poor city of Houston witnessed this firsthand in 2017 as we lived through the brutal Hurricane Harvey. The ground could not absorb the pounding, relentless rainfall and thousands of people were flooded out of their homes. To compensate, the city had to intentionally flood some neighborhoods to take the pressure off the dams and more lives were devastated. This is similar to what can occur in your liver. As the state of microbiome dysregulation becomes worse, inflammation will no longer be controlled, and your liver function tests will rise to abnormal levels. As you realign your health, they will normalize again.

 DO

1. **Eat fiber.** The microbiome is fed by the fibers of plant foods. We used to think fiber was just for bowel movement motility, but we now understand that those

fibers are also feeding the good guys in our gut! Each gut species has a preferred food source, so plant diversity in the diet is super important. If you only eat a few vegetables or the same vegetables day after day, you will only feed one or two species and starve the others. Aim for six different vegetables every day. It's also helpful to eat at least one vegetable from the following categories per day:

- **Green leafy veggies**, which include kale, bok choy, collard greens, swiss chard, dandelion greens, spinach and arugula

- **Cruciferous veggies**, such as broccoli, cauliflower, brussels sprouts and cabbage;

- **Root vegetables,** such as turnips, beets, parsnips, carrots and jicama, and sunchokes.

Certain fruits, such as deep-colored berries, are also super high in fiber and can be eaten once per day or so to help strengthen the microbiome.

2. **Eat starch.** New research is showing the importance of resistant starch for the gut. Resistant starch is unable to be broken down for digestion and moves through the GI tract intact. This makes it the perfect food for your gut bugs that feed on this starch and create short-chain fatty acids that are good for the brain and your gut. Resistant starch has shown to be helpful in the prevention of colon cancer and insulin resistance, seems to help the body burn fat, and can improve sleep.

Because resistant starches are resistant to digestion, they can cause bloating and gas, especially in someone who is prone to these conditions to start with. The best way to incorporate these in the diet is to start low and slow. Some examples of resistant starch are as follows: green bananas, raw plantains and plantain flour, white rice cooked in water and coconut oil and then cooled (the resistant starch forms in the cooling process), potatoes cooked and then cooled, and potato starch.

Designs for Health recently created a fiber supplement with resistant starch made from potato starch and green bananas and is a great place to start because you can start by adding a very small amount into smoothies or just dissolve it in water.

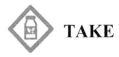 **TAKE**

1. Probiotics/Spores
If you have a delicate GI system, start with the probiotics instead of the spores. Then we recommend rotating between regular probiotics and spores every 4–6 months.

Probiotics
We need to respect and support the trillions of bacteria that live in our gut. While all females have about 99% similar DNA, our microbiomes differ by about 35%. As no test is perfect in telling us exactly our bacterial makeup at any one time, we want to do everything we can to support a healthy microbiome. The ancient practice of playing in the dirt helped us establish a healthy microbiome. As outdoor activity has been widely replaced by indoor time, we do not get our hands as dirty anymore. Although obtaining our microbes through nature is preferred, supplementation can somewhat bridge the gap.

The original probiotic was made using the typical bacteria found in cow gut. It was somewhere to start and something we could study years ago when today's technology was in its infancy. Capsules were thin and needed to be refrigerated to keep the bacteria alive. While some companies still use a thin capsule, many have developed a way to keep their probiotics alive at room temperature. Today, most probiotics will contain *Lactobacillus* and *Bifidobacter* species in colony-forming units anywhere from 5 billion to 25 billion. Because of the low pH of stomach acid, it is often best to take your probiotics away from your meals.

Ortho Molecular, Designs for Health, Xymogen, and Klaire Labs all make very good probiotics. It is also a good idea to rotate your probiotics every 6 months.

Fermented foods and beverages are a great source of natural probiotics. A few examples are sauerkraut, kimchi and other fermented veggies, and kombucha. These foods are made from live bacterial cultures or yeast and are easy to digest. Don't confuse these foods with pickled foods. Pickled foods have been preserved in an acidic medium, often vinegar. While vinegar itself is produced from a fermentation process, these pickled foods don't contain the live probiotics and enzymes that fermented foods do (although they are often still delicious and nutritious).

Fermented foods made from live cultures will be in the refrigerated section of the store and have a fresh, but somewhat sour, taste. You can adapt to the taste by mixing 1 tbsp. of fermented veggies with a serving of fresh ones.

Kombucha is an example of a fermented beverage and has gained much popularity over the last few years. There is a large amount of variety in the quality of kombucha available on the market. Kombucha that has been fermented for an appropriate amount of time should taste somewhat bitter and not sweet (sugar is required to ferment the tea used to brew kombucha but should be consumed by the live culture in the process) and contain 5 g of sugar or less per serving on the bottle. Be aware that most bottles of kombucha contain 2 servings, not 1, of the bubbly beverage.

Making your own yogurt or kombucha is a very cost-friendly way to get high doses of probiotics. Homemade yogurt can contain about 700 billion beneficial bacteria compared to the 15–25 billion in a typical probiotic supplement. Check out Cultures for Health online for everything you need to make your own ferments at home.

Spores
Scientists have long thought that spores may be a huge contributor to the health of our microbiome. They have a strong outercoat that could survive any harsh climates. Some of their benefits are as follows:

- Evaluate the gut surroundings and balance what is in the large intestine already. We call this *quorum sensing*.

- Decrease inflammation in the gut. Less inflammation here will enable estriol to be produced in the gut while minimizing inflammation in the blood. Remember that inflammation and inflammatory cells in the blood will affect nerve cells, including the brain.

- Support gut lining and minimize intestinal permeability.

Spores enter your GI tract and really start to clean up, sometimes to the point that you have very bad constipation and do not feel good. I call this the Poor Man's Stool Test. If you take spores and this happens, it is a good sign that your gut needs help. A milder probiotic in the above category, a GI map test, and a visit to your functional medicine practitioner should be on your list.

2. Vitamin K2
Vitamin D will not pair with calcium to make our bones strong unless vitamin K2 is present. Vitamin K2 is produced by a healthy, diverse microbiome; that is the primary way we obtain our daily allowance. It is found also in abundance in natto, which is fermented soybeans made using the bacteria *Bacillus subtillis*. Because the smell of natto has often been described as sweaty feet, old cheese, warm garbage, etc., it is not a very popular food in the US. Vitamin K2 can also be found in goose liver, egg yolks, dark chicken meat, and grass-fed butter.

Most pharmaceutical grade vitamin D3 supplements contain some vitamin K2, usually about 10 mcg of K2 for each 1,000 IU of vitamin D. This combination is safe and actually beneficial in pregnancy. Using micronutrient testing will help you get some idea if you are deficient and need higher levels of supplementation. Dr. Kiran Krishnan of Microbiome Labs believes that most people in the US are deficient in vitamin K2. He recommends regular K2 supplementation because of our typical diet; 150–300 mcg is recommended.

3. Colostrum/IgG capsules

Colostrum is a premilk fluid produced in the mammary glands of mammals that have recently given birth. It is also used for boosting the immune system, healing injuries, repairing nervous system damage, improving mood, and contributing to an overall sense of well-being as it supports production of balanced neurotransmitters in a healthy microbiome. A natural agent for killing bacteria and fungi, colostrum is a great supplement for gut healing and repair.

IgG is an immunoglobulin concentrate supplement derived from colostrum. Usually the concentration of the IgG is more potent than what is found in colostrum. Most pharmaceutical grade supplements contain natural immunoglobulins with bioactive proteins, and growth factors. These components support immune function, healthy inflammation control, gut barrier function, and gastrointestinal health and tissue repair. Think of it as a street sweeper moving through your intestine and cleaning up.

This more concentrated formula is usually used after being treated to rebalance the microbiome. Orthomolecular IgG Protect is a good option here. You can take this every day during your first month on the Roadmap and then three times a week after that.

4. Bone Broth/Collagen Peptides

Bone Broth

Bone broth is sought out by people around the world to deal with a wide variety of health issues and to maximize longevity. According to Chris Masterjohn, PhD, eating nose to tail is one of the best ways to maintain optimal weight, gut, and overall health. This process enables us to extract all of the important parts of the animal that enhance us and to pay homage and respect to the animals that nourish us.

Bones and connective tissue are storehouses for essential amino acids and minerals, which are lacking in many diets today. While often not feasible to eat whole bones or tissue, you can still enjoy these health benefits by sipping bone broth. Sipping ¼ to ½ cup daily provides nourishment for the gut, skin, hair, and mind. Collagen and all of the other mentioned components are extracted when you simmer bones for a long period of time, especially with an apple cider vinegar medium.

Typically, the longer bone broth simmers, the more collagen you'll extract. You can use the bones of any healthy animal to make bone broth depending on your taste; bone broth made from cows does tend to have a stronger taste than chicken.

Making your own bone broth is easy and economical, and many great recipes are available online. We also have a recipe available on our website at www.dianginsbergMD.com when you download our free detox guide. If you are local to Texas, Yonderway Farm in Fayetteville is a great source for bones and/or bone broth that is already made; they ship anywhere in Texas. Their website is www.yonderwayfarm.com.

Collagen Peptides
Collagen peptides are the building blocks of bone broth and are instrumental in renewing tissues, such as bones, joints, and even skin. They are easier to consume than bone broth as you can buy them in a powder and add them to any drink. Collagen peptides act as a type of messenger to trigger the synthesis and reorganization of new collagen fibers at the cellular level. They are bioavailable and ready to assimilate into GI tissues and immediately begin to help heal our gut.

While bone broth contains collagen, it is at times a bit cumbersome to consume, and many do not like the taste. Ortho Molecular, Designs for Health, and Vital Proteins all make great convenient collagen supplements.

One thing to be aware of with collagen: If you are prone to anxiety, collagen may increase your anxiety. Most of these reports are anecdotal, but tryptophan depletion may be to blame. If this occurs, adding 5-htp supplementation, which is a form of the amino acid tryptophan, may help. However, often the best thing is to decrease the amount of collagen or eliminate it altogether.

Collagen may also aggravate migraines in susceptible individuals so proceed with caution.

DRAW

While measuring our precise levels of light e~
following tests can be a good indicator of circadian rhythm. It is ~~~~
for these tests to be done by a saliva sample.

Four-Point Cortisol
Cortisol should be highest in the morning to wake you up and then
slowly decrease throughout the day to its lowest level before bedtime.
Irregular patterns of cortisol indicate disruptions in your circadian
rhythm.

Melatonin (Waking/Midday/2 am)
Melatonin should also follow a pattern with levels rising sharply around
9 pm and staying elevated for about 12 hours. Upon waking, levels will
start to fall and should be almost nondetectable midday.

 DO

1. Have early sun in your eyes. Watching the sun rise or enabling early
sun to activate the receptors in your eyes is one of the most important
things you can do for yourself every day. This act is one of the biggest
reconnections to our environment that we have lost. Dr. Jack Kruse has
an excellent article on his blog about this very subject, and he is an
excellent resource to strengthen your mitochondria and to help you
utilize light to strengthen your brain function and energy levels.

Even 10–15 minutes in the morning of watching the sun rise will help.
For optimal vitamin D levels, aim for sun exposure around noon, with
minimal clothing for 15–30 minutes.

If you have to be at work before the sun rises, especially in the winter
months, you can still get that morning sun by leaving your desk for a

utes and walking outside. Your mood and productivity will be
uch better after doing this for a week that your boss couldn't
ssibly object!

2. Use blue light blockers for computer/office work during the day and red lights at home in the evening. While people often associate blue light with phone screens, it can also come from fluorescent light and LED light. Blue light from sunlight to welcome the day is wonderful; it is the constant blue light from the computer screen that is an issue. Blue light at the wrong times from the wrong sources has been linked to sleep dysfunction as it can delay the release of melatonin. Eventually this will cause a disruption in the body's circadian rhythm, which can then lead to leptin resistance. The hard work that goes into adopting a clean diet to reverse PCOS may be done in vain if the light/dark melatonin cycle is out of sync.

Red lights are best as we head into evening. Actual sleeping should be done in total darkness. Black-out curtains may be necessary for the bedroom.

The blue light blockers come in all shapes and sizes. Ra Optics is the brand recommended by many of the experts. Red light can be used in a simple screw bulb and can be found at most home improvement stores. Sleep Ready is a lightbulb created specifically to emit light wavelengths that promote sleep and can be found on Amazon. If you want to explore the healing aspects of red light, you can invest in a Joovv light, which many experts recommend for skin issues, athletic performance, joint pain, and more.

3. Meditate. Meditation at the start of the day is an additional support for good cortisol patterns. Ten to fifteen minutes of meditation before you get out of bed will quiet your mind and help prevent that big cortisol spike in the morning and the crash that often accompanies it.

Meditation seems daunting at first, and most of us struggle to sit quietly and just be. But there are many YouTube videos, apps, and books that help with learning this process. A simple search on YouTube for meditation to reduce stress, anxiety, etc., will yield lots of useful results. A good additional tool for those who need guided meditation is the MUSE Headband. It is very simple to use; it reads the calming waves in your brain and transmits the response to your cellphone. The app speaks to you using your own headphones on how to relax your mind. What is really cool about this product is that, when you are doing it correctly, you will hear birds, but if your mind starts to spin, you will hear waves crashing. A calm voice reminds you to gently slow your breathing and relax.

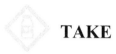 **TAKE**

1. Melatonin
The dosing and timing of this supplement are very important.

Melatonin is a hormone secreted by the pineal gland and is involved in the regulation of the human sleep-wake cycle and circadian rhythm. Melatonin is released into the bloodstream exclusively at night, following the circadian rhythm. Mechanistically, natural melatonin levels start to increase approximately 2 hours before natural sleep onset and peak approximately 5 hours later. Should circadian cycles become dysregulated, the secretion of melatonin will become dysregulated. Again, while there is no substitute for natural light cycles, adding melatonin at sleep time can help restore sleep. Melatonin supplements can effectively help treat sleep disruption caused by this dysregulation by mimicking the natural endogenous melatonin. It will bind to the same receptors and activate the same downstream pathways.

Remember that it *does* matter when you take melatonin. Melatonin taken in the middle of the day can move your biological clock up, while melatonin taken in the middle of the night can move it forward. If you have trouble falling asleep, you should take it in the evening, about 30 minutes to 1 hour before bedtime.

People who wake in the middle of the night and cannot fall back to sleep may have a different issue of insomnia. Melatonin will not help this. We then recommend using 200 mg of theanine before you go to bed. This is not a circadian rhythm problem but more of a neurotransmitter problem. Realignment of your neurotransmitters is discussed in Chapter 5 on microbiome.

If you have symptoms of advanced sleep phase syndrome, in which there is a strong desire to fall asleep and wake up several hours too early, some suggest taking melatonin in the morning upon waking. However, there is no real medical literature that supports this concept.

You should also ensure that you have ample light exposure at the opposite time—morning or night—from when you take melatonin. This is especially important for night owls.

While melatonin is safe, high levels are just not necessary. A study conducted by MIT in 2001 states that 0.3 mg of melatonin is sufficient to restore peaceful sleep in adults. Usually between 0.5 and 3 mg is a good dose to help you rest.

2. Adaptogenic Herbs

Adaptogenic herbs help modulate cortisol by altering the response of the cell to cortisol signaling. While cortisol is yelling at the cell to activate and make adrenaline and glucose to fight the "tiger," the adaptogenic herbs tell the cell to chill. They actually mimic the feeling of moderate exercise—that overall stable, healthy, refreshed feeling you have after a long brisk walk in lovely cool weather. This overtakes the dramatic cortisol response and results in good balance.

While nothing replaces sunlight and reconnecting with your environment, trying to modulate your cortisol so your body does not always read a stress signal is optimizing your health. Remember that adaptogenic herbs are different from vitamins and can be pretty powerful. Consulting with an Ayurvedic or Chinese medicine practitioner can be helpful when considering supplementation of these herbs. Below are a few examples:

Ashwaganda. This is probably the most well-known of the bunch. Human studies have shown that it can decrease anxiety, C-reactive protein and cortisol. 3–6 g daily is recommended.

Bacopa monnieri. This herb is recognized for its ability to reduce anxiety and improve cognitive function. Studies have shown that it can reduce physiological stress, especially when taken before the stressful event (such as when studying for finals, an upcoming presentation, or visiting the in-laws!). 300 mg daily is recommended.

Cordyceps. Mice studies have shown that *Cordyceps* can increase energy and reduce oxidative stress. It may also enhance athletic performance, especially in older adults. 300 mg, once to three times daily, was given in the studies.

Holy basil. Evidence supporting its use for lowering anxiety and stress and increasing libido has made this herb a favorite among many. It may also help increase muscle mass, but the jury is still out on that one. There is one negative mark against this herb—some studies indicate that it may decrease male fertility, possibly due to its high urolic acid content. 500 mg twice daily is recommended.

Mucuna pruriens. This herb contains large amounts of the precursor to the neurotransmitter dopamine to help improve focus and attention. It may also lower stress, anxiety, and depression and improve fertility in men. 100–200 mg daily is recommended.

Panax ginseng. There are many different forms of *Panax ginseng*, but red and white are the most popular forms. It can increase the sense of well-being and improve cognition and focus by reducing fatigue, and some studies show that it may reduce blood sugar in otherwise healthy individuals. 200 mg daily is recommended.

Rhodiola rosea. The right amount of this can reduce exhaustion and fatigue but too much may actually increase these issues. It may also reduce C-reactive protein; however, this effect was mostly seen after a bout of exhaustive exercise. 200 mg twice daily seems to be a safe place to start.

If you like to experiment, then trying your own combination is fine; see what works. Apex Energetics's Adaptocrine, Designs for Health's Catecholacalm, and Xymogen's Adrenal Essence are some of our favorite combination adaptogenic supplements.

5) EMF - *Electromagnetic Force and it's disruption of both our Mitochondrial Energy Production and Life's Building Blocks (External Environment interacting with the Internal)*

 DRAW

EMF can be highly disruptive to your melatonin production and, as discussed previously, any disruptions in your melatonin production will result in poor sleep. Melatonin is a powerful hormone and antioxidant, and lowered or disrupted levels lead to the following:

- **Less Rapid Eye Movement (REM) Sleep.** REM sleep stimulates the brain regions used in learning. Like deep sleep, REM sleep is associated with increased production of proteins. The frontal cortex is the part of the brain that interprets information from the environment during waking hours. Random signals from the brain stem during REM sleep enable the cortex to create a "story" out of fragmented brain activity.

- **Less Optimal Detoxification.** In deep sleep, your body removes many of its toxins.

- **Less Healing.** In deep REM sleep, the body recovers from the breakdown of the day.

- **Decreased Brain Function, Poor Memory, and Focus.** While we sleep, the electric charge circulating around our brain is off-loaded into the gray matter. This process happens also when we meditate. No conscious thoughts coming in enables the system to actually recharge for optimal function the next day. Without rejuvenating sleep, brain function is compromised in every way.

Obtain the following:
- Salivary melatonin levels at 7 am, noon, and 3 am to be sure your curve is optimal.
- SpectraCell's MNT test, as described in the Energy Balance section, contains an area called SPECTROX. It is a measure of your antioxidant defense status.

DO

Grounding/Earthing

How do you ground? It is very simple; you have most likely done this action many times, especially as a young child playing outside! Walk barefoot in the grass, sand, or local dirt path. Your body is a conductive surface, and the earth's energy flows through it. Wood, asphalt, vinyl, and especially carpeting are not good at enabling the flow of energy. Grounding to the soil aids in good electrical and blood flow throughout our body. This can help decrease red blood cell (RBC) aggregation and blood clot formation. Earth's surface is a global electrical circuit. This circuit has three main generators:

- The sun's rays that transmit charged particles

- The ionospheric wind, or the upper atmosphere containing charged particles broken apart by the sun's strong energy. When the sun is active, more and more charged particles are created!

- Thunderstorms, which are continually active around the globe with thousands of bolts of lightning that strike the earth per minute. This creates a constant current and negative charge to the surface of the earth.

As the soil's electrons are conducted to the human body, the grounded body heals. Inflammation calms, circadian rhythms regulate, and sleep and cortisol patterns improve. Within 2 seconds of simple, direct contact with the ground, such as walking barefoot or sitting or lying down on the soil's surface, benefits begin.

Barefoot substitutes consist of specific mats, bands, and sheets, which when connected to a specific home or office outlet connects you to the earth's energy. This process is done via the ground wire of the outlets, and you must be very careful. If your outlet is connected to a dirty electric source or the current is problematic, you will be doing more harm than good.

The mat at Earthing comes highly recommended by many and they have a whole site of products that you can try (https://www.earthing.com/).

TriField EMF Meter/Coronet Meter

You can try this device to evaluate the EMF load in your home.

I must credit what I've learned about EMF to Nicolas Pineault and his book *The Non-Tinfoil Guide to EMFs*. You can purchase it online, and it is a wonderful tool. Please read his book and follow his recommendations. Using the TriField Meter, I checked the EMF load in my home and was pleased that overall the load was low. I do have dimmer/flicker switches on many of my wall sockets that I addressed with products from GreenWave (www.greenwavefilters.com)

A Few More Things You Can Address

Simply start with creating distance between your body and the source of EMFs. A fascinating fact is that placing as little as 1 ft between you and your EMF-emitting device reduces EMF exposure by 80%; 2 ft or more reduces that number to nearly 95%.

- Place your cell phone on airplane mode when you sleep and keep it away from your head. When in active use, either use the speaker with the phone 1 ft away as you speak or use an old-fashioned cord earphone to connect instead of the Bluetooth connection.

- Keep your laptop off your lap. *Time Magazine* published an article indicating that laptop use can contribute to infertility when kept on your lap. Although we don't have a definitive answer on this one, we do know that EMF waves can interfere with DNA and our reproductive DNA is important. Keep your laptop on the table or desk as much as possible when you work.

- Invest in a defender shield for your device. Nick Pineault does say that a defender shield (www.defendershield.com) will work to some extent. However, the EMF leaves the computer from all angles. Getting a standing or laptop desk can remove 95% of this issue and also keep you from sitting all day.

- Use an ethernet cable to plug directly into the wall. It helps eliminate the need for Wi-Fi if you are not using it.
- Turn off your Wi-Fi at night or whenever you are not using it. You can use a simple timer purchased at your local hardware store; it is the same timer that turns your holiday lights on and off. You plug your router into the timer and then the timer into the wall. The Wi-Fi will turn off and on again at the time you set so you do not have to think about it.

- Invest in an EMF harmonizer to neutralize the effects of harmful radiation and radio and electromagnetic frequencies that are emitted by our electronic devices. Here are some of the recommended types:
  o Geoclense® Home and Workplace Harmonizer
  o EarthPulse™ pulsed electromagnetic field devices
  Some are very expensive and not necessarily better so do your research before purchasing.

- Certain plants can absorb some of this ionizing radiation like they absorb sunlight, which they convert into sugars and food. They add calm green to your space while increasing oxygen levels. EMFs from your computer will bounce all around your room, and the plants will help absorb some of them. While more research needs to be done, these plants are easy to care for, do well indoors, and can be kept in smaller pots while adding a healthy breath of life! Below are some examples.

Cacti and Succulents
Cacti and succulents are perfect plants as they are cute and very simple to take care of. They are not only hardy plants that thrive in almost any environment, but NASA researchers discovered that these plants are great for absorbing certain types of EMF radiation. You only need to water these about once per week, and they should be kept by a window for optimal sun.

The Snake or Airplane Plant
The real name for this plant is *Sansevieria*. You might see these plants in large pots where they can flourish and grow tall, but they can also be put in smaller pots for the desk.

They are often seen decorating an office or desk. Water once a week or when the top inch of soil feels dry, always allowing water to drain. Never allow the soil to become saturated. Keep in low, medium, or bright light.

Aloe vera

This is the perfect desk plant—it's small and a great producer of essential oils as well as a powerful air purifier. Also a succulent, *Aloe vera* is already known for robust growth in challenging environments. *Aloe* has well-known healing properties for sunburns caused by ultraviolet radiation. Its air purifying properties make it effective for absorbing radiation in the air, bouncing off your walls, or any other type being emitted by electronic devices. Water well once a week; give the soil a good soaking. It also loves the sunlight.

The Narcissus Plant

Adorned with beautiful flowers, the Narcissus plant is also very efficient at converting ionizing ultraviolet radiation into plant food. It is a beautiful decoration that can aid in greater health. Water once or twice a week but keep in a well-drained soil. It can live in full sun to partial shade.

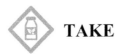 **TAKE**

Whole Foods

EMF will increase your overall free-radical production and weaken the enzymes that help neutralize them. Should your testing show you need antioxidant support or you want to add some antioxidants to your regimen, remember that the best source is FOOD. Green leafy vegetables and other nonstarchy vegetables that are varied in type and color are the best prime source. You cannot supplement your way out of a good diet. Folate or B9 is an extremely beneficial antioxidant for EMF support and is best obtained from green leafy vegetables. Vitamin E is also important for antioxidant support and can be found in sunflower seeds, almonds, green leafy veggies, and pumpkin. Using functional nutrient testing can help guide your diet and supplementation if needed.

Designs for Health's Ultimate Antioxidant Full Spectrum is my recommended supplement for poor antioxidant status.

Balancing the neurotransmitters GABA and norepinephrine is very important. As EMF can disrupt the electrical force within us, sleep and anxiety can increase. This is described brilliantly in the text *The Schumann Resonance*, detailing how the calming pulse of the earth correlates with our meditative brain waves. When the frequency of the earth is elevated, anxiety and overall neurotransmitter disruption is also elevated. This is described often as anxiety that just comes out of nowhere with no specific reason behind it.

Designs for Health's Liposomal Neurocalm can be taken for general anxiety at any time or in the evening to help you settle down before bedtime.

Apex's Adaptocrine contains adaptogenic herbs and can be taken up to three times a day as needed for your own personal calming.

Essential Oils
Essential oils could be added at any point in the Roadmap—the benefits of essential oils are endless! These oils can aid in any area where support is needed and can interact with your body in a number of positive ways. When applied to your skin, they are absorbed quickly. Applying certain oils to different areas of the body can create different intended effects. Inhaling the aromas from essential oils can stimulate areas of your brain that affect emotions, behaviors, anxiety, sleep, relaxation, and long-term memory.

As different parts of the brain play a role in controlling some unconscious physiological functions, such as breathing, heart rate, and blood pressure, we often see that essential oils can exert a physical effect on your body in a positive way. Massages using these essential oils have been shown to reduce anxiety, depression, and reduce stimulation of the sympathetic (fight or flight) nervous system.

Be careful that you obtain your oil from a truly reputable company to ensure they are pure and clean. We use Young Living Essential Oils in our office (www.youngliving.com). Young Living has created a technique called the Raindrop Technique Massage that is super relaxing and good for the immune system. It is something I love to do before taking a long plane ride. You can find a certified massage therapist in your area who performs this kind of massage by searching the database of alternative practitioners: https://www.alternativesforhealing.com/find-a-practitioner/.

6) Hormones

 DRAW

These are suggested labs that you can ask your practitioner to evaluate for you, but please proceed with caution on this particular part of the Roadmap. **If you only evaluate hormone levels and address those with hormone replacement, you will often get deeper into trouble.** What I often see in my office is that patients do not want to address their diet or blood sugar dysregulation but simply want to add a hormone cream or pill and get better. However, the Roadmap is very specific in that all the lanes must be traveled together.

Keep in mind that the "normal" range for any lab comes from patient averages. These patients are often medical students whose average age is somewhere between twenty-two and twenty-eight. Academic universities may also recruit patients that are at "optimal health" and use their numbers as the norms. Because of our bioindividuality, it can be tough to know exactly what should be normal for you, but these labs can give us a general idea and at least provide a baseline number when treatment protocols are initiated.

Drawing hormone labs when you are on the birth control pill will not reflect your true state of being. Some labs such as for sex hormone binding globulin (SHBG) can be altered by the birth control pill for up to a year. For an accurate assessment, it is best to be off the birth control pill for 3–6 months before drawing hormone labs. Here are some recommended labs and what they may mean:

Estradiol
Best method of testing: For PCOS, it is helpful to look at estradiol in blood. Looking at estradiol in saliva is a second step if there is still no normalization of the menstrual cycle after the initial metabolic state is fixed.

What it means: When blood sugar is dysregulated, your estradiol will be at steady state and may be *elevated* even though you don't have periods. It also may be very low. If you are not having regular cycles but your estradiol levels are above 80 pg/dL, this is often a sign that dysregulated blood sugar is a contributing factor and should be addressed before hormone therapy is initiated.

Estrone
Best method of testing: Saliva on day 19, 20, or 21 of your cycle if you are having regular cycles. If not having regular cycles, the collection can be done on any day that you are not bleeding.

What it means: High levels of estrone indicate that your body cannot get rid of excess estrogen. This could mean that your liver and the ability to off-load extra hormones and most likely toxins are part of your problem. Looking at how to detox and then maintain this on a daily basis is the key to health here. This process is covered in the DO part of this section.

Progesterone
Best method of testing: Saliva on day 19, 20, or 21 of your cycle if you are having regular cycles. If not having regular cycles, the collection can be done on any day that you are not bleeding.

I often see patients that have had their progesterone checked at some random time in their cycle whether regular or irregular. It is usually low, and the patient is given supplementation. Adding progesterone before fixing all the other components will add to insulin resistance and you will gain weight.

What it means: Be careful, as the lab result may not actually be very significant! Blood progesterone levels are only significant when looking at pregnancy support. Normal values in nonpregnant women have a wide range throughout the second half of your cycle and cannot indicate whether you need supplementation or not. Even saliva testing must be evaluated carefully. Different saliva labs use different methods. Some labs use an enzyme test and look at all the progesterone and by-products, while others look at only the pure molecule in a centrifuge-type system. I do not want to write a whole chapter and bore you on lab testing here, but just understand that you must be careful with the lab result you use and make sure it is interpreted by a functional medicine practitioner who clearly understands hormone and metabolic balance. In our practice, progesterone supplementation is mostly used in those women who have completed all the other parts of the Roadmap but still struggle with cycle-related sleep, anxiety, or spotting issues.

Sex Hormone Binding Globulin
Best method of testing: Blood

What it means: It is very important to address SHBG because this is a big key to glucose metabolism balance. This topic is covered in detail in Chapter 3. SHBG controls how many of your total hormones are bound up and unusable and how many are floating free to enter into the cells and send signals. SHBG also controls the natural balance of fatty acids and glucose that is ever so important in nature. An SHBG level below 35 nmol/L is very low and a sign of blood glucose and fatty acid dysregulation.

Remember that birth control pills contain high doses of estradiol and will cause SHBG to be falsely elevated. This abnormality can persist up to a year after the pills are stopped.

Total and Free Testosterone/DHEA
Best method of testing: Blood, but saliva can also be used

What it means: High levels of total (bound and unbound) testosterone indicate PCOS. Normal total testosterone levels in women range from 8 to 60 ng/dL. As SHBG decreases, the amount of free testosterone increases. While lab values of 0.06–4 ng/dL are considered normal, free testosterone levels above 1 ng/dL indicate the need to have your glucose/insulin and overall metabolic state carefully evaluated. Elevated testosterone is part of PCOS and does seem to have a genetic component. However, if you consider your environment, both inside and outside the body, you can normalize these values *despite* your genetics.

Values of DHEA-S (the sulfated compound is what is measured in blood) generally run in blood optimally between 100 and 350 µg/dL. These levels will go up as total testosterone elevates, and these two hormones will often convert back and forth. Tissue levels of both can be checked through the saliva. Testosterone is a big molecule and generally has a difficult time making its way into the saliva. So if you see elevated levels there, then your body has shifted too far into the male hormone production. You will often see elevated DHEA for the same reason, although they both do not have to be elevated to indicate dysfunction.

Fasting Insulin and Insulin 1 and 2 Hours after Eating
These hormones are also covered in the first section of the Roadmap on Energy Balance.

Best method of testing: Blood

What it means: Fasting insulin levels should be around 7 µIU/mL. Higher levels indicate dysregulated blood sugar that can lead to excess fat storage. It is often difficult to draw insulin levels 1–2 hours after eating, but it is a very useful way of deciphering blood sugar regulation. Ideally, insulin levels should peak 30 min to 1 hour after eating and then slowly decrease. A disruption in this pattern indicates insulin resistance. The second-hour insulin should be below 50.

Fasting Glucose and Glucose 2 Hours after Eating
Best method of testing: Blood

What it means: High fasting glucose (90 mg/dL or above) indicates blood sugar dysregulation. Fasting readings below 70 mg/dL also indicate hypoglycemia, which is a state of dysregulation. Glucose 2 hours after eating should be between 90 and 115 mg/dL. Glucose that is higher than this after a meal can indicate a meal that was too high in refined carbs or carbs that are not right for your bioindividuality.

Leptin
Best method of testing: Blood

What it means: Leptin is a hormone that is made in fat cells. It sends feedback to the brain when fat storage is full so that the brain can send satiety signals to dampen hunger. While levels above 25 ng/mL can define leptin resistance on the lab sheet, once leptin starts to creep over 15 ng/mL, signs of leptin resistance such as body shape changes and weight loss resistance, start to appear. At this point, weight gain will occur more easily, and you will feel more frustrated as you try to make diet changes. Remember it is diet, lifestyle, light, and circadian rhythm issues that create leptin issues. Leptin resistance eventually can also affect estrogen secretion and fertility.

Follicle Stimulating Hormone and Luteinizing Hormone
Best and only method of testing: Blood

What it means: The traditional definition of PCOS states that the luteinizing and follicle stimulating hormones are in a 3:1 ratio with elevated estradiol levels. The reasoning behind this value stems from the dysregulated "pulse" of male hormones (androgens/testosterone/DHEA) into the central nervous system as the young female reproductive system is developing. This is generally the cause of irregular cycles in girls when they first start their cycle. I see many women who claim they had normal menses as a child, which could indicate a genetic predisposition to develop PCOS less, and working on the steps outlined in the Roadmap can reverse the syndrome. Use this ratio as a marker for change that will be visibly seen as you adopt the changes outlined in the Roadmap.

Pregnenolone
Best and only method of testing: Blood

What it means: Vitamin B5 plus healthy levels of cholesterol (at least 160) plus carbon chains will produce the mother hormone pregnenolone. Pregnenolone will sacrifice everything to make cortisol for your fight or flight response. A normal level should be 50–151 ng/dL. Levels below 50 ng/dL can indicate you are either struggling to make pregnenolone owing to low cholesterol levels and/or bad digestion, or the

More detox ideas can be downloaded from dianginsbergMD.com in a free detox guide.

Avoid Toxic Exposure to Xenoestrogens
Environmental xenoestrogens are substances including certain drugs, pesticides, and industrial by-products that can negatively affect your hormones. High levels of estrogens that come from outside your body are associated with harmful effects as these can mimic the hormones that your body produces hormones and interfere with your endocrine system. These are collectively called endocrine disruptors. Unfortunately, xenoestrogens exert their effects through binding and activation of estrogen receptors, similar to your own natural estrogen hormone. However, endocrine disruptors can often affect hormones (sometimes in opposite directions) of the same endocrine pathway. This process can create harmful effects on human health.

Here are some of the biggest offenders:

1. **Tap water**
   Unfortunately, much of our water is contaminated with petroleum derivatives—the primary source of xenoestrogens. Drink filtered water whenever possible. We have a Berkey filter and dispenser (www.berkeywaterfilter.com) at home and our office, and the difference in taste is remarkable!

2. **Phthalates**
   Soft plastics used as packaging materials and that compose your favorite bottled water are often treated with this particular chemical compound. Invest in a good glass water bottle. Unfortunately, the plastic wrap covering the food in the premade section of the store contains some of the highest xenoestrogen levels. If you have to heat food in the microwave, invest in glass containers and cover it with a moist paper towel, not plastic. Avoid Styrofoam cups and plastic containers—use glass containers whenever possible!

3. **Commercially raised meat and dairy products**
   These products are often contaminated with growth hormones to help make them bigger and more valuable on the market. This

process will expose us to a significant amount of xenoestrogens. Try to consume hormone-free, grass-fed, and humanely raised animal products whenever you can. Not only will this support your endocrine system, but it is much better for the environment and supports local business. If you are in Texas, check out Yonderway Farm for an awesome selection of grass-fed and pastured meats and eggs, along with local treasures from the surrounding community. Raw dairy farms are growing in Texas and around the country as well. US Wellness Meats also has a good selection for those that are not local to Texas.

4. **Anything that contains insecticide or pesticide residues**
Another reason to eat local, organic foods whenever possible.

5. **Parabens**
A type of preservative first introduced in the 1950s, parabens are used to prolong shelf life in many health and beauty products by preventing the growth of mold and bacteria within them. Studies have shown that some of these parabens will mimic the activity of the hormone estrogen in the body's cells. Parabens have even been found present in breast tumors.

Many of the xenoestrogens enter through the skin and go directly to tissue. Therefore, they do not pass through the liver for detoxification. As they are completely absorbed by the body, they can be up ten times more potent and destructive than those consumed orally.

6. **Foods that contain soy proteins**
Soy protein foods can be packed with condensed, unnaturally high amounts of estrogen. Soy isoflavones bind to estrogen receptors and can produce either weak estrogenic or antiestrogenic activity. The components of soy can disrupt hormones by slipping into the estrogen hormone receptor on the cell and mimicking what estrogen would have done in the cell. But since it doesn't fit the receptor exactly, the message gets distorted and can be dangerous. The only way we recommend eating soy is if it's fermented into natto or miso.

7. **Disposable menstrual products**
   In conventional tampons, the FDA has detected dioxins, a class of chemical contaminants that may increase our health risk. Synthetic tampons and sanitary napkins also may contain chlorine, fragrance, wax, surfactants, and rayon. Use feminine products made with natural materials instead. Specific examples include LOLA, Natracare, Cora, and Organyc.

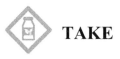 **TAKE**

Maca
The multifunctional effect of Maca on endocrine relationships may explain why it is reported in the literature as a positive regulator of hormones in the body. It is particularly helpful in women struggling to keep their balance optimal and a perfect addition to the patient with PCOS who is doing everything right but still struggling with hormone optimization. The suggested standard dose is 1,500–3,000 mg.

Diindolylmethane
Diindolylmethane (DIM) is a compound that occurs when cruciferous vegetables arrive in the stomach and are digested. DIM restores healthy hormone balance. Working with your healthy microbiome, it converts estrogens that need to be detoxified into benign estrogen metabolites. This way, it aids in hormone balance and cancer protection. In food form, it's found in cruciferous veggies like broccoli. Most reputable supplement companies have a version of it.

Vitamin C/Quercetin/Rutin (Flavonoids)
Patients with PCOS usually have issues with antioxidant balance, which can lead to infertility, endometriosis, and heavy or dysfunctional menstruation. Flavonoids are phytonutrients found in almost all fruit and veggies, and they have a healing effect on many of the unwanted medical consequences of PCOS. Flavonoids have a variety of biological actions including antimicrobial, antiviral, anti-inflammatory, antioxidant, liver protective, and lipid-lowering activities.

Quercetin is instrumental in balancing adiponectin levels, while studies have shown that vitamin C can minimize free radicals and boost progesterone levels. Rutin is a specific bioflavonoid, which is necessary for the absorption of vitamin C and has a noteworthy range of scavenging characteristics on oxidizing species. Designs for Health's C+Biofizz is one of our favorite vitamin C supplements because it contains quercetin and rutin and comes in a great-tasting powder that mixes easily with water; ¼ tsp. once or twice per day is a good starting dose.

Saw Palmetto

Saw palmetto is a low-growing palm tree grown in the West Indies and in coastal regions of the southeastern United States. While this plant is generally regarded as beneficial to men, it has some therapeutic value for women as well. Saw palmetto is available in tablet, capsule, tea, and natural berry forms. Experts are not entirely clear on exactly how saw palmetto influences hormones but speculate that saw palmetto may block the enzyme that turns testosterone into dihydrotestosterone (DHT). It is this converted substance that sits on the cell receptors and creates all the male or androgenic effects in PCOS. Stopping the conversion of testosterone into DHT minimizes acne and hirsutism and aids in the return of normal menstrual cycles.

The suggested standard dose is 400-mg capsule/day or 1 tsp. liquid extract/day, post meal.

Warning: Do not take saw palmetto if you are on the birth control pill.

Berberine

Berberine is a bioactive compound that can be extracted from a group of shrubs called *Berberis*. It is as a potent insulin sensitizer. Berberine has been shown to improve insulin resistance in a similar fashion to metformin. The benefits of berberine have been directly compared to metformin's in women with PCOS. It is found in the cells of various organs, including the heart, brain, and muscle, which further clarify the major role it seems to have in regulating metabolism.

Clinical studies have evaluated berberine HCl at different dosages ranging from 500 to 1,500 mg per day, for as long as 6 months in adults. The most common dosage appears to be 1,500 mg a day. These should be taken in three divided doses with meals.

Zinc

While zinc is not the first supplement to come to mind in PCOS, it has been shown to have a significant impact owing to its role in glucose regulation. Not only is zinc very important in the mitochondria to maximize energy generation from burning fat, but it is also of ultimate importance in the glucose utilization cycle. Numerous laboratory studies show that zinc supplementation can reduce fasting glucose and improve insulin functioning in animal models. While studies in humans are a bit more limited, evidence shows that humans can benefit from taking zinc. Zinc supplementation results often in improved insulin function and blood sugar control.

In general, zinc is best absorbed on an empty stomach but does seem to cause nausea when taken without food, which causes quite a dilemma. It's best to start with a low dosage, about 5–10 mg, to see how well it's tolerated. Too much zinc may cause a copper deficiency, so sometimes it's best to take these supplements together. An ideal dosage would be about 25 mg per day.

Calcium-D-Glucurate

This compound removes harmful estrogens and estrogen metabolites responsible for many unpleasant conditions such as fibrocystic breasts, breast lumps, estrogen-receptor-positive breast cancers, endometriosis, menstrual headaches, mood swings, and premenstrual syndrome (PMS). Calcium-D-glucurate is produced by combining glucaric acid with calcium and works by helping to conjugate or bind these estrogens and aiding in their removal in the intestines.

The suggested standard dose is 500–1,000 mg.

Essential Oils—Progessence Plus

Progessence™ Plus, a blend from Young Living, is designed specifically for women. It contains USP progesterone (United States Pharmacopeia, meaning the product was produced in accordance with good manufacturing practices) from wild yam extract, vitamin E, and other essential oils like frankincense, bergamot, and peppermint. At times when hormones are dysregulated, this combination seems to modulate or calm the see-saw to create a feeling of physical and mental hormonal balance.

The recommended standard dose is two to four drops per day on the back of the neck or forearms in the evening.

28-Day PCOS Environmental Reset

Hopefully by this point in the book, you have read all the fun science of PCOS and understand (and love!) your body a little more. Now it's time to put this new knowledge into action. Below are the guidelines for the 28-Day PCOS Environmental Reset. These guidelines were created to help your body sync its internal and external environments to maximize its natural state of being.

- Eat 6–9 cups of vegetables daily. A serving equals about ½ cup of any vegetable besides leafy greens; 1 serving of leafy greens equals 1 cup. Remember that your gut microbiome depends on the diversity of your plant foods so try to choose three to four different vegetables daily. If you are prone to gas and bloating, increasing your vegetable intake may make that issue worse. In that case, eat your vegetables cooked instead of raw and try to minimize high FODMAP veggies. FODMAP stands for fermentable oligo-, di-, mono-saccardies, and polyols and represents a group of carbohydrates that can cause gas, bloating and general discomfort in certain people with irritable bowel syndrome (IBS) and other gut issues. High FODMAP vegetables are indicated by the # symbol in the following tables. These high FODMAP vegetables are very nutrient dense and should only be restricted for a short time while you work on healing the gut.

Table 1. Vegetables by category (try to choose a variety of vegetables each day and at least one from each category)

Green Leafy Vegetables	Cruciferous/Allum Vegetables	Colorful/Root Vegetables
All forms of kale	Broccoli/Broccolini/Broccoli rabe#	Beets
Dandelion greens	Cauliflower (all colors)#	Carrots
Turnip greens	Cabbage (all colors)#	Parsnips
Bok choy	Brussel sprouts	All squash (butternut, summer, winter, spaghetti, etc.)
Swiss chard (green and red)	Watercress	Cucumber
Arugula	Turnips	Jicama
Spinach	Garlic#	Jerusalem artichoke (sunchoke)
Collard greens	Onions (all types)#	Artichoke#
Mustard greens	Radishes (all types including Daikon)	Ginger
Mizuna	Rutabaga	Bell peppers*
Endive	Kohlrabi	Tomato*#
Beet greens	Horseradish	Eggplant*
Romaine	Asparagus#	Green beans
Radicchio#	Leek#	Celery#
	Shallot#	Mushrooms#
		Okra

These are nightshade vegetables and are fine for most, but if you have excess inflammation or an autoimmune condition, avoiding these may be necessary for recovery.

- Experiment with adding 1–3 servings of starchy vegetables, legumes, or grains daily. The need for more carbohydrates (the vegetables listed in Table 1 are mostly carbohydrate) is very individual, but in our practice, we have found that many women do best when they add 1 serving of starch at lunch and 1–2 servings at dinner.

A serving size of a starch is about ½ cup. Do not include gluten-containing grains such as wheat or farro during this 28-day period. Examples of the recommended starches are in Table 2. Again, the high FODMAP starches are represented with the # symbol.

Table 2. Starchy vegetables, gluten-free grains, and legumes

Gluten-Free Grains (these are best digested if soaked overnight or sprouted)	Legumes (these are best digested if soaked overnight or sprouted)	Starchy Vegetables
Rice (all types)	Lentils (all types)#	White, red, or purple potatoes*
Steel-cut oats	Black beans#	Sweet potato or yam
Quinoa	Chickpeas#	Yucca
Corn (organic only)	Pinto beans#	Water chestnut
Amaranth	Green peas#	Taro
Millet	Lima beans#	Plantain
Teff		Pumpkin

*Nightshade

- Include 1–2 servings of fruit per day (optional). Serving sizes are written next to each fruit below. Fruit should be local and in season when possible; remember that we are trying to re-sync your body with the natural circadian rhythm of life. It is best to choose fruits that are deep in color throughout the fruit such as berries, pomegranates, citrus fruits, cherries, etc., owing to their high antioxidant content. Table 3 represents the seasons of various fruits in America.

Table 3. Fruits by season, with serving size

Winter	Spring	Summer	Fall
Apples (4 oz)	Apples	Apples	Apples
Bananas (3 oz)	Apricots (2 small)	Apricots	Bananas
Grapefruit (½ medium)	Bananas	Bananas	Cranberries (¼ cup)
Kiwi (1 fruit)	Kiwi	Blackberries (1 cup)	Grapes (½ cup)
Lemons/limes	Lemon/lime	Blueberries (1 cup)	Kiwi
Oranges (½ medium)	Pineapple	Cantaloupe (1 slice)	Lemon/lime
Pears (4 oz)	Strawberry (1 ¼ cup	Cherries (⅔ cup)	Mangos
Pineapple (¼ cup)		Honeydew melon (1 slice)	Pears
		Lemons/limes	Pineapple
		Mango (¼ cup)	Raspberries
		Peaches (3 oz)	
		Plums (2 small)	
		Raspberries (1 cup)	
		Strawberries	
		Watermelon (1 cup)	

- Include 3–4 oz of protein at each meal. The examples in Table 4 are all animal-based proteins. While we respect the heart that goes behind the choice to be a vegetarian, we have found in our practice that rebalancing the PCOS system is extremely difficult on a vegetarian diet. If you are a vegetarian, you can rely somewhat on starchy legumes such as those listed in Table 3, but keep in mind that those foods are more carbohydrate than protein. Soy is often a vegetarian protein of choice, but soy in the US is very genetically modified and often hard to digest, so we only recommend fermented soy such as tempeh or natto. Try to incorporate fish at least twice per week.

Table 4. Proteins

Meat/Eggs	Seafood
Whole Eggs (the actual protein is in the white, but the yolk is important for hormone balance)	All shellfish (as local as possible)
Grass-fed beef (all cuts)	Wild caught Alaskan salmon
Pasture-raised chicken (including the skin and all cuts	Mackerel
Pasture-raised duck or other fowl	Sardines
Game meat like venison	Anchovies
Pasture-raised pork	Tuna (among the higher-mercury fish, so only consume about once per week)
	Pacific cod
	Redfish

It is recommended to buy your meat, eggs, and seafood from a local farmer/fisherman when possible. These small farms tend to be good stewards of the land and the animal by rotating the animals to revive the farmland and allowing the animal to live in humane conditions that cause the animal to thrive in good health. When these animals are fed their native diet (not gummy bears and other candy that often is fed to feedlot animals to make them fatter), they do not cause the flatulence and methane gas issues that feedlot animals do. Their meat is also richer and more nutrient dense, giving you more bang for your buck. If local to Texas, check out Yonderway Farm in Fayetteville; they deliver all over Texas (www.yonderwayfarm.com). If you live elsewhere, check out US Wellness Meats (www.grasslandbeef.com) or The Weston A. Price Foundation (www.westonaprice.org) for a list of farms near you. Vital Choice (www.vitalchoice.com) or Sea to Table (www.sea2table.com) are good resources for wild caught fish.

- Include 1–2 servings of healthy fats at each meal. These fats will help you feel more satisfied with your meals and help stabilize the blood sugar rollercoaster. They also make the food taste so much better! The fats recommended below are those that do not promote inflammation in the body. The serving size for most cooking oils is 1 tbsp. Other serving sizes are listed in Table 5, as well as their smoke points.

Table 5. Healthy fats, with their smoke points and serving size

High-Heat Cooking Fats	Low Heat or No Heat	No Heat or Whole Foods
Ghee (450)	Olive oil (325)	Flaxseed oil (should be kept in fridge)
Pasture-raised lard (370)	MCT oil (325)	Olives (20 large, pitted)
Pasture-raised duck fat (375)	Full-fat coconut milk (¼ cup)	Avocado (½ medium)
Pasture-raised beef tallow (420)		All nuts and seeds and nut/seed butter, except peanuts (which should be avoided during reset). Keep to 2 handfuls or 2 tbsp. per day. Avoid any nut/seed butters with added sugars.
Butter (350)		Shredded coconut (½ cup)
Coconut oil (350)		
Avocado oil (375)		
Sesame Oil (350)		

- Include one to two superfoods per day for maximum health. Superfoods are nutrient-dense foods that are outside the norm of most American diets and tend to offer more benefits as far as gut health, trace minerals, or detoxification support. Starting with 1 tbsp. per day and increasing to about ¼ to ½ cup will take you far on your health journey. The following are some examples of nutritional superfoods:
  - Bone broth (recipe can be found at dianginsbergMD.com, included in the free detoxification guide
  - Fermented vegetables such as sauerkraut or kimchi

- Sea vegetables such as dulse, nori, or seaweed
- Fermented cabbage juice such as Gut Shot by Farmhouse Cultures
- Water or coconut kefir with less than 5 g of sugar per serving
- Kombucha (plain or with less than 5 g of remaining sugar per serving
- Liver or other organ meats

- The following foods should be eliminated during the 28 days:
  - All sugar with the exception of stevia. Because of the important immune and antimicrobial properties of honey, 2 ½ tsp per day are allowed but be aware that honey is a high FODMAP food.
  - All flour, including almond and coconut flour and other gluten free flours. Foods broken down into flour raise blood sugar much quicker than that food in its whole form.
  - All gluten-containing foods
  - Peanuts
  - Avoid cooking with or using the following oils as salad dressings: canola, peanut, vegetable, corn, shortening, sunflower, and safflower oils, margarine
  - Soy with the exception of fermented soy
  - Alcohol
  - All dairy except for ghee or butter

Dairy is a complete food, having a good combination of fats, protein, and carbohydrates. However, there are a few issues with the typical woman with PCOS. Low-fat dairy is chosen by most women due to the mistaken notion that eating fat leads to being fat. Low-fat dairy has been shown to rapidly raise blood glucose levels, making it a poor choice for those with PCOS. But even full-fat dairy has some drawbacks, though. Most of the cows in America are casein A1 cows, which is a hybrid of the European casein A2 cows. These A1 cows tend to produce more milk and be somewhat heartier. However, the protein they produce in their milk is highly allergenic (hence the rapid increase in dairy allergies in this country) and inflammatory to the gut lining. This is the main reason it is eliminated during this 28-day period. A2 cows are bred in the US but mostly on small family farms. If you can find milk, or the products made from these A2 cows in your area, it can be a healthy addition to your diet, especially in its raw, unpasteurized form. Right now, in most states, this milk is either totally unavailable or available only directly from small family farms. However, keep in mind that dairy does contain insulin-like growth factors, and if you find that adding dairy back to your diet has caused the return of some unwanted symptoms, it is best to eliminate it completely.

- Try fasting once or twice per week. If your blood sugar is very dysregulated or you have a serious endocrine condition such as type 1 diabetes, fasting will not be an option for you. However, the majority of women with PCOS can benefit greatly from it. There are so many different ways to do this, but the main goal is the same—spend some significant time without food. The easiest way to try this is to stop eating around 5–6 pm and don't eat again until 8 am or so the next day. That gives you a good 14 to 16-hour window without food coming into the system. One of the advantages of eating this early is it puts you in a position to go to bed with low insulin, allowing the body to hear the leptin signal while sleeping. If the 14 to 16-hour fast goes well, incorporating it 2–3 times per week can really help some women regulate their hormones. Some women even do well fasting for a full 24 hours once per week or so. The key is that fasting should ultimately make you feel better (more energy, better sleep, more mental clarity) even if you feel hungry. If fasting makes you feel very weak or foggy brained or disrupts your sleep, your body simply isn't ready for this step yet.

- Start the day with 10 minutes of sun exposure. You can go outside and read the paper, take a short walk, or simply stand in the sun. If you leave for work before the sun comes up, simply walk outside as soon as the sun comes up wherever you are and take that 10 minutes to recharge before officially starting the day.

- Go for a 10 to 15-minute walk outside at lunchtime daily.

- Invest in blue light blockers for your office and home. Wear them at the office during long intervals of continuous computer work and wear them at home while watching TV or utilizing electronic devices.

- Don't use any electronic devices after 8 pm.

- Turn off your Wi-Fi at night, and keep your electronic devices outside of your bedroom. If you need your phone in your bedroom, turn it to airplane mode.

- Exercise daily. If you haven't exercised in a while, make a goal to walk, swim, or bike daily for 20–30 minutes during this 28-day period. If you are already doing consistent cardio exercise, add in high-intensity interval or weight training two to three times per week. Finding a good personal trainer or fitness coach can be super helpful in navigating proper weight-lifting techniques, especially in the beginning.

- On our YouTube channel (dianginsbergMD), we have posted lots of different workouts that can be done from home with minimal equipment.

- Add yoga one to two times per week. Many free videos can be found on YouTube.

- Take an Epsom salt bath two to three times per week. For extra detox support, you can use the following recipe:

Clay Detox Bath
½ cup bentonite clay
½ cup Epsom salts
Essential oils if desired

Dissolve the Epsom salts in a warm/hot bath and add essential oils if desired. For the clay, choose *one* of the following two options:

  1. Vigorously mix the clay in to a small amount of water until the clumps are mostly dissolved. Do not use metal

for this! I mix with a plastic spoon in a glass jar. Add the clay mix to the bath and soak for at least 20 minutes.

2. Mix the clay with a small amount of water to make a paste. Stand in the tub full of water and rub the clay mix all over your body to create a skin mask and let dry for 5 minutes before sitting down. This provides direct contact with the skin and effectively pulls toxins from the skin. Soak in a bath for at least 20 minutes or as long as desired. While soaking, use a washcloth to scrub any remaining clay off the skin.

- Buy a cactus or *Aloe vera* for your desk and your home. See the EMF section of the Roadmap for more details on plants that can reduce your EMF load.

- Meditate daily for 10–20 minutes. Great free options are available on YouTube and Headspace. You can find meditation guides for anxiety, sleep issues, overall stress management, and more.

- The following supplements are optional but may optimize your experience on the 28-day reset. It is best to check with your doctor first before starting any new supplements. You do not need to take all of these supplements, just pick one or two from the list:

  1. **Myo/chiro-inositol** balanced in a 40:1 ratio. This is especially helpful if your cycles are irregular. Our favorite is Designs for Health's Sensitol. Take 2 capsules twice daily.

  2. **Berberine**. Take 400 mg daily

  3. **CM Core** by Orthomolecular. This product contains berberine and alpha lipoic acid, which has shown to be a powerful combination for blood sugar management. The prescribed dose is 1 capsule three times daily. You do not need to take extra berberine if you take this product.

4. **Metabolic Synergy** by Designs for Health. This multivitamin and mineral formula contains alpha lipoic acid, chromium, and other vitamins, minerals, and antioxidants for healthy glucose regulation. The prescribed dosage is 2 capsules three times per day.

5. **Omega-3 fish oil**. Take 1,000 mg daily of mixed EPA and DHA.

Afterword

The world of medicine is sometimes slow to change so it may be hard to find a medical doctor that is willing to think outside the box and offer other treatment methods for PCOS besides birth control, spironolactone and metformin. Even if your current allopathic physician is willing to draw some of the more functional labs, they may not be able to help you interpret these labs with a mindset of using nutritional and lifestyle-based therapies. Under our current insurance model of care, physicians must see a certain number of people each day just to keep the lights on and the staff paid. This model generally allows around 15 minutes maximum per patient, and current surveys show that the average patient gets around 7.5 minutes with their doctor. To sit down and look at the root cause of your irregular cycles, infertility, irregular bleeding, or hair loss means spending much more than the allotted 15 minutes. On top of this, most doctors know that these symptoms are likely to resolve, at least in the short run, with birth control or any combination of spironolactone and metformin. Even if the patient doesn't ultimately feel her best on this combo of meds, the symptoms the patient came to see the doctor about would somewhat resolve so doctors feel this equates to success. But this approach is equivalent to putting a piece of tape over the check engine light without taking the car in for repairs.

Functional medicine is an area of medicine that is focused on the root cause of underlying disease. Many medical doctors are becoming certified in functional medicine and The Institute of Functional Medicine has a listing of certified practitioners on https://www.ifm.org/find-a-practitioner/. The Metabolic Medical Institute also certifies practitioners in functional medicine (Dr. Ginsberg is board certified through the Institute in Anti-Aging and Regenerative Medicine), and a search of their practitioner database would also be helpful: https://www.a4m.com/find-a-doctor.html.

Working with a naturopath or nutritional therapy practitioner can also be helpful as they will really help you implement practical diet and lifestyle changes, and they can often work with you on a more long-term basis for accountability. Nutritional therapy practitioners (NTP) are certified under the Nutritional Therapy Association and are trained in using real food to correct nutritional deficiencies that may lead to imbalance anywhere in the body. Many of these practitioners have established relationships with medical professionals where the medical professional will order the necessary labs, interpret them, and create a treatment protocol that will be fleshed out by the NTP for increased patient success. You can find a list of NTPs in your area at www.nutritionaltherapy.com.

References

Chapter 2

Guangchang, Pang, Junbo Xie, Qingsen Chen, and Zhihe Hu. "Energy Intake, Metabolic Homeostasis, and Human Health." *Food Science and Human Wellness* 3, no. 3–4 (September/December 2014): 89–103, https://doi.org/10.1016/j.fshw.2015.01.001.

Wang, Rui, and Ben Willem J. Mol "Rotterdam Criteria for Polycystic Ovary Syndrome: Evidence-Based Criteria?" *Human Reproduction* 33, no. 2 (February 2017): 261–64, https://doi.org/10.1093/humrep/dew287.

Chapter 3

Carlomagno, Gianfranco, et al. "The D-CHIRO-Inositol Paradox in the Ovary." *Fertility and Sterility* 95, no. 8 (June 2011): 2515–16, https://doi.org/10.1016/j.fertnstert.2011.05.027.

Deswal, R., et al. "Sex Hormone Binding Globulin—An Important Biomarker for Predicting PCOS Risk: A Systematic Review and Meta-Analysis." *Current Neurology and Neuroscience Reports*, U.S. National Library of Medicine, February 2018.

Genazzani, Alessandro D. "Inositol as Putative Integrative Treatment for PCOS." *Reproductive BioMedicine Online* 33, no. 6 (December 2016): 770–80, https://doi.org/10.1016/j.rbmo.2016.08.024.

Genazzani, Alessandro D., et al. "Effects of a Combination of Alpha Lipoic Acid and Myo-Inositol on Insulin Dynamics in Overweight/Obese Patients with PCOS. *Endocrinology and Metabolic Syndrome* 3, no. 3 (October 2014): 1000140, https://doi.org/10.4172/2161-1017.1000140.

Guangchang, Pang, Junbo Xie, Qingsen Chen, and Zhihe Hu. "Energy Intake, Metabolic Homeostasis, and Human Health." *Food Science and Human Wellness* 3, no. 3–4 (September/December 2014): 89–103, https://doi.org/10.1016/j.fshw.2015.01.001.

Kalra, B., S. Kalra, and J.B. Sharma. "The Inositols and Polycystic Ovary Syndrome." *Indian Journal of Endocrinology and Metabolism* 20, no. 5 (2016):720–724.

Sortino, M. A., S. Salomone, M. O. Carruba, and F. Drago. "Polycystic Ovary Syndrome: Insights into the Therapeutic Approach with Inositols." *Front Pharmacology* 8 (June 2017): 341, https://doi.org/10.3389/fphar.2017.00341.

Pintaudi, B., G. Di Vieste, and M. Bonomo. "The Effectiveness of Myo-Inositol and D-Chiro Inositol Treatment in Type 2 Diabetes." *International Journal of Endocrinology* 2016 (2016): 9132052.

Unfer, Vittorio, et al. "Effects of Inositol(s) in Women with PCOS: A Systematic Review of Randomized Controlled Trials." *International Journal of Endocrinology* 2016 (2016), https://doi.org/10.1155/2016/1849162.

Chapter 4

Asayama, Kohtaro, et al. "Decrease in Serum Adiponectin Level Due to Obesity and Visceral Fat Accumulation in Children." *Obesity Research* 11, no. 9 (September 2003): 1072–79, https://doi.org/10.1038/oby.2003.147.

Bahreini, Mehdi, et al. "The Effect of Omega-3 on Circulating Adiponectin in Adults with Type 2 Diabetes Mellitus: A Systematic Review and Meta-Analysis of Randomized Controlled Trials." *Canadian Journal of Diabetes* 42, no. 5 (October 2018): 553–59.

Ciampelli, Mario, et al. "Impact of Insulin and Body Mass Index on Metabolic and Endocrine Variables in Polycystic Ovary Syndrome." *Metabolism–Clinical and Experimental* 48, no. 2 (February 1999): 167–72

Ciaraldi, Theodore P., et al. "Polycystic Ovary Syndrome Is Associated with Tissue-Specific Differences in Insulin Resistance." *Journal of Clinical Endocrinology and Metabolism* 94, no. 1 (2008): 157–63.

Cezaretto, Adriana, et al. "Association of Adiponectin with Cognitive Function Precedes Overt Diabetes in the Brazilian Longitudinal Study of Adult Health: ELSA." *Diabetology and Metabolic Syndrome* 10, no. 54 (July 2018): https://doi.org/10.1186/s13098-018-0354-1.

Deswal, R., et al. "Sex Hormone Binding Globulin—An Important Biomarker for Predicting PCOS Risk: A Systematic Review and Meta-Analysis." *Current Neurology and Neuroscience Reports*, U.S. National Library of Medicine, February 2018.

Kadowaki, Takashi, and Toshimasa Yamauchi. "Adiponectin and Adiponectin Receptors." *Endocrine Reviews* 26, no. 3 (May 2005): 439–51.

Kirstein, M., et al. "Advanced Protein Glycosylation Induces Transendothelial Human Monocyte Chemotaxis and Secretion of Platelet-Derived Growth Factor: Role in Vascular Disease of Diabetes and Aging." *Proceedings of the National Academy of Sciences of the United States of America* 87, no. 22 (1990): 9010–14.

Mostowik, Magdalena, et al. "Omega-3 Polyunsaturated Fatty Acids Increase Plasma Adiponectin to Leptin Ratio in Stable Coronary Artery Disease." *Cardiovascular Drugs and Therapy* 27, no. 4 (2013): 289–95.

Ng, Roy Chun-Laam, and Koon-Ho Chan. "Potential Neuroprotective Effects of Adiponectin in Alzheimer's Disease." *International Journal of Molecular Sciences* 18, no. 3 (March 2017): 592, https://doi.org/10.3390/ijms18030592.

Pizzini, Alex et al. "The Role of Omega-3 Fatty Acids in Reverse Cholesterol Transport: A Review." *Nutrients* 9, no. 10 (October 2017): 1099, https://doi.org/10.3390/nu9101099.

Woodward, Lavinia, et al. "Unravelling the Adiponectin Paradox: Novel Roles of Adiponectin in the Regulation of Cardiovascular Disease." *British Journal of Pharmacology* 174, no. 22 (2016): 4007–20.

Yang, Kailin, et al. "Effectiveness of Omega-3 Fatty Acid for Polycystic Ovary Syndrome: A Systematic Review and Meta-Analysis." *Reproductive Biology and Endocrinology* 16, no. 1 (March 2018): https://doi.org/10.1186/s12958-018-0346-x.

Chapter 5

"Alcohol: Balancing Risks and Benefits." *The Nutrition Source*, February 2019. https://www.hsph.harvard.edu/nutritionsource/healthy-drinks/drinks-to-consume-in-moderation/alcohol-full-story/.

Canani, Roberto Berni, et al. "Potential Beneficial Effects of Butyrate in Intestinal and Extraintestinal Diseases." *World Journal of Gastroenterology* 17, no. 12 (2011): 1519–28.

Diamanti-Kandarakis, Evanthia, Charikleia Christakou, and Evangelos Marinakis. "Phenotypes and Enviromental Factors: Their Influence in PCOS." *Current Pharmaceutical Design* 18 no. 3 (January 2012): 270–82.

Engen, Phillip A., et al. "The Gastrointestinal Microbiome: Alcohol Effects on the Composition of Intestinal Microbiota." *Alcohol Research: Current Reviews* 37, no. 2 (2015): 223–36.

Foster, Jane A., et al. "Stress and the Gut-Brain Axis: Regulation by the Microbiome." *Neurobiology of Stress* 7 (March 2017): 124–36.

Galley, Jeffrey D., et al. "Exposure to a Social Stressor Disrupts the Community Structure of the Colonic Mucosa-Associated Microbiota." *BMC Microbiology* 14, no. 189 (July 2014): https://doi.org/10.1186/1471-2180-14-189.

Gluecka, C. J., et al. "Incidence and Treatment of Metabolic Syndrome in Newly Referred Women with Confirmed Polycystic Ovarian Syndrome." *Metabolism* 52, no. 7 (July 2003): 908–15.

Guilliams, Thomas G., and Lena Edwards. "Chronic Stress and the HPA Axis: Clinical Assessment and Therapeutic Considerations." *The Standard* 9, no. 2 (2010): http://www.pointinstitute.org/wp-content/uploads/2012/10/standard_v_9.2_hpa_axis.pdf

Lammers, Karen M., et al. "Translational Chemistry Meets Gluten-Related Disorders." *Chemistry Open* 7, no. 3 (February 2018): 217–32, https://doi.org/10.1002/open.201700197.

Leonard, Maureen M., et al. "Celiac Disease and Nonceliac Gluten Sensitivity: A Review." *JAMA* 318, no. 7 (2017): 647–56, https://doi.org/10.1001/jama.2017.9730.

Lowe, Patrick P., et al. "Alcohol-Related Changes in the Intestinal Microbiome Influence Neutrophil Infiltration, Inflammation and Steatosis in Early Alcoholic Hepatitis in Mice." *PLoS One* 12, no. 3 (March 2017): e0174544, https://doi.org/10.1371/journal.pone.0174544.

Liu, Lu, and Gang Zhu. "Gut-Brain Axis and Mood Disorder." *Frontiers in Psychiatry* 9, no. 223 (May 2018), https://doi.org/10.3389/fpsyt.2018.00223.

Mutlu, Ece, et al. "Intestinal Dysbiosis: A Possible Mechanism of Alcohol-Induced Endotoxemia and Alcoholic Steatohepatitis in Rats." *Alcoholism: Clinical and Experimental Research* 33, no. 10 (2009): 1836–46, https://doi.org/10.1371/journal.pone.0174544.

Queipo-Ortuño, María Isabel, et al. "Influence of Red Wine Polyphenols and Ethanol on the Gut Microbiota Ecology and Biochemical Biomarkers." *American Journal of Clinical Nutrition* 95, no. 6, (June 2012): 1323–34.

Rosenbaum, Michael, Rob Knight, and Rudolph L. Leibel. "The Gut Microbiota in Human Energy Homeostasis and Obesity." *Trends in Endocrinology and Metabolism* 26, no. 9 (2015): 493–01, https://doi.org/10.1016/j.tem.2015.07.002.

Samsel, Anthony, and Stephanie Seneff. "Glyphosate Pathways to Modern Diseases. II: Celiac Sprue and Gluten Intolerance." *Interdisciplinary Toxicology* 6, no. 4 (2013): 159–84, https://doi.org/10.2478/intox-2013-0026.

Sudo, Nobuyuki, et al. "Postnatal Microbial Colonization Programs the Hypothalamic-Pituitary-Adrenal System for Stress Response in Mice." *Journal of Physiology* 558, no. 1 (2004): 263–75.

Voigt, Robin M., et al. "Circadian Disruption: Potential Implications in Inflammatory and Metabolic Diseases Associated with Alcohol." *Alcohol Research: Current Reviews* 35, no. 1 (2013): 87–96.

Zinöcker, Marit K., and Inge A. Lindseth. "The Western Diet-Microbiome-Host Interaction and Its Role in Metabolic Disease." *Nutrients* 10, no. 3 (March 2018): 365.

Chapter 6

Arvind Babu, K., et al. "CYP1A1, GSTM1 and GSTT1 Genetic Polymorphism Is Associated with Susceptibility to Polycystic Ovaries in South Indian Women." *Reproductive BioMedicine Online* 9, no. 2 (August 2004): 194–00.

Guilherme, Victor, et al. "Vitamin D Receptor Polymorphisms and the Polycystic Ovary Syndrome: A Systematic Review." *Journal of Obstetrics and Gynaecology Research* 43, no. 3 (March 2017): 436–46, https://doi.org/10.1111/jog.13250.

He, Chunla, et al. "Serum Vitamin D Levels and Polycystic Ovary syndrome: A Systematic Review and Meta-Analysis." *Nutrients* 7, no. 6 (June 2015): 4555–77.

Matosin, Natalie, Cristiana Cruceanu, and Elisabeth B. Binder. "Preclinical and Clinical Evidence of DNA Methylation Changes in Response to Trauma and Chronic Stress." *Chronic Stress* 1 (February 2017), https://doi.org/10.1177/2470547017710764.

Chapter 7

Ahima, Rexford S., and Daniel A. Antwi. "Brain Regulation of Appetite and Satiety." *Endocrinology and Metabolism Clinics of North America* 37, no. 4 (2008): 811–23, https://doi.org/10.1016/j.ecl.2008.08.005.

Kiefer, Florian W. "The Significance of Beige and Brown Fat in Humans." *Endocrine Connections* 6, no. 5 (2017): R70–79, https://doi.org/10.1530/EC-17-0037.

Klok, M. D., S. Jakobsdottir, and M. L. Drent. "The Role of Leptin and Ghrelin in the Regulation of Food Intake and Body Weight in Humans: A Review." *Obesity Reviews* 8, no. 1, (January 2007): 21–34, https://doi.org/10.1111/j.1467-789X.2006.00270.x.

Nieminen, Petteri. "Survival of the Fattest—Leptin, Melatonin, Thyroxine and the Seasonal Adaptation of Mammals." PhD dissertation, University of Joensuu, 2010.

Reneau, James, et al. "Effect of Adiposity on Tissue-Specific Adiponectin Secretion." *PloS One* 13, no. 6 (June 2018): e0198889, https://doi.org/10.1371/journal.pone.0198889.

Riddle, Misty, et al. "Insulin Resistance in Cavefish as an Adaptation to a Nutrient-Limited Environment." *Nature* 555 (March 2018): 647–651, https://doi.org/10.1038/nature26136.

Chapter 8

Ben-Hamo, Miriam, et al. "Circadian Forced Desynchrony of the Master Clock Leads to Phenotypic Manifestation of Depression in Rats." *eNeuro* 3, no. 6 (December 2016): 1–13, https://doi.org/10.1523/ENEURO.0237-16.2016.

Borer, Katarina T. "Counterregulation of Insulin By Leptin As Key Component of Autonomic Regulation of Body Weight." *World Journal of Diabetes* 5, no. 5 (October 2014): 606–29, https://doi.org/10.4239/wjd.v5.i5.606.

Challet, E. "Keeping Circadian Time with Hormones." *Diabetes, Obesity and Metabolism* 17, no. S1 (September 2015): https://doi.org/10.1111/dom.12516.

Dibner, Charna, and Frédéric Gachon. "Circadian Dysfunction and Obesity: Is Leptin the Missing Link?" *Cell Metabolism* 22, no. 3 (September 2015): 359–60, https://doi.org/10.1016/j.cmet.2015.08.008.

Gerhart-Hines, Zachary, and Mitchell A. Lazar. "Circadian Metabolism in the Light of Evolution." *Endocrine Reviews* 36, no. 3 (June 2015): 289–304, https://doi.org/10.1210/er.2015-1007.

Kettner, Nicole M et al. "Circadian Dysfunction Induces Leptin Resistance in Mice." *Cell Metabolism* 22, no. 3 (September 2015): 448–59, https://doi.org/10.1016/j.cmet.2015.06.005.

Mohawk, Jennifer A., Carla B. Green, and Joseph S. Takahasi. "Central and Peripheral Circadian Clocks in Mammals." *Annual Review of Neuroscience* 35 (July 2012): 445–62, https://doi.org/10.1146/annurev-neuro-060909-153128.

Nilsson, Dan E. "Eye Evolution and Its Functional Basis." *Visual Neuroscience* 30, no. 1/2 (2013): 5–20.

Takahashi, Joseph S. "Circadian-Clock Regulation of Gene Expression." *Current Opinion in Genetics and Development* 3, no. 2 (1993): 301–09.

Yılmaz, Setenay Arzu, et al. "The Relationship between Polycystic Ovary Syndrome and Vitamin D Levels." *Turkish Journal of Obstetrics and Gynecology* 12, no. 1 (March 2015): 18–24, https://doi.org/10.4274/tjod.76148.

Chapter 9

Environmental Health Trust. "National Toxicology Program Finds Cell Phone Radiation Induces DNA Damage." Accessed April 17, 2019. https://ehtrust.org/national-toxicology-program-finds-cell-phone-radiation-induces-dna-damage/

EMF Solutions. "Mold Produces 600 Times More Bio-Toxins with EMF." Accessed April 17, 2019. https://emfsol.com/mold-produces-600-times-more-bio-toxins-with-emf/

Cardis, E., and M. Hatch. "The Chernobyl Accident—An Epidemiological Perspective." *Clinical Oncology* 23, no. 4 (May 2011): 251–60, https://doi.org/10.1016/j.clon.2011.01.510.

Ghaly, M. et al. "The Biologic Effects of Grounding the Human Body During Sleep as Measured by Cortisol Levels and Subjective Reporting of Sleep, Pain, and Stress."

Journal of Alternative and Complementary Medicine 10, no. 5 (October 2004):767–76, https://doi.org/10.1089/acm.2004.10.767.

Havas, Magda. "Dirty Electricity Elevates Blood Sugar among Electrically Sensitive Diabetics and May Explain Brittle Diabetes." *Electromagnetic Biology and Medicine* 27, no. 2 (July 2009): 135–46, https://doi.org/10.1080/15368370802072075.

JRS ECO Wireless. "EU Reflex Study Shows DNA Damage Caused by Radiation from Wireless Devices and Mobile Phones." Accessed April 17, 2019. https://www.jrseco.com/eu-reflex-study-shows-dna-damage-caused-by-radiation-from-wireless-devices-and-mobile-phones/?c=cf13ce20305c.

Kıvrak, Elfide Gizem, et al. "Effects of Electromagnetic Fields Exposure on the Antioxidant Defense System." *Journal of Microscopy and Ultrastructure* 5, no. 4 (2017): 167–76, https://doi.org/10.1016/j.jmau.2017.07.003.

Lane, Nick. *Life Ascending: The Ten Great Inventions of Evolution.* New York: W.W. Norton, 2010.

Lansdown, A., and D. Aled Rees. "The Sympathetic Nervous System in Polycystic Ovary Syndrome: A Novel Therapeutic Target?" *Clinical Endocrinology* 77, no. 6 (December 2012): 791–01, https://doi.org/10.1111/cen.12003.

Lin, Kang-Wei, Chuan-Jun Yang, Hui-Yong Lian, and Peng Cai. "Exposure of ELF-EMF and RF-EMF Increase the Rate of Glucose Transport and TCA Cycle in Budding Yeast" *Frontiers in Microbiology* 7, no. 1378 (August 2016): https://doi.org/10.3389/fmicb.2016.01378.

Milham, Samuel. "Evidence That Dirty Electricity Is Causing the Worldwide Epidemics of Obesity and Diabetes." *Electromagnetic Biology and Medicine* 33, no. 1 (June 2013): 75–78, https://doi.org/10.3109/15368378.2013.783853.

National Institute of Environmental Health Sciences. "Electric and Magnetic Fields." Accessed April 17, 2019. https://www.niehs.nih.gov/health/topics/agents/emf/index.cfm.

Oschman, J. L., G. Chevalier G, and R. Brown. "The Effects of Grounding (Earthing) on Inflammation, the Immune Response, Wound Healing, and Prevention and Treatment of Chronic Inflammatory and Autoimmune Diseases." *Journal of Inflammation Research* 8 (March 2015): 83–96, https://doi.org/10.2147/JIR.S69656.

Pineault, Nicolas. *The Non-Tinfoil Guide to EMFs: How to Fix Our Stupid Use of Technology.* CreateSpace Independent Publishing Platform, 2017.

Saroka, Kevin S et al. "Similar Spectral Power Densities Within the Schumann Resonance and a Large Population of Quantitative Electroencephalographic Profiles: Supportive Evidence for Koenig and Pobachenko." *PloS One* 11, no. 1 (January 2016): e0146595, https://doi.org/10.1371/journal.pone.0146595.

Yakamenko, I., et al. "Low Intensity Radiofrequency Radiation: A New Oxidant for Living Cells." *Oxidants and Antioxidants in Medical Science* 3, no. 1 (2014):1–3, https://doi.org/10.5455/oams.240314.ed.002.

Chapter 10

An, Y. et al. "The Use of Berberine for Women with Polycystic Ovary Syndrome Undergoing IVF Treatment." *Clinical Endocrinology* 80, no. 3 (March 2014): 425–31, https://doi.org/10.1111/cen.12294.

Arentz, Susan, et al. "Combined Lifestyle and Herbal Medicine in Overweight Women with Polycystic Ovary Syndrome (PCOS): A Randomized Controlled Trial." *Phytotherapy Research* 31, no. 9 (2017): 1330–40, https://doi.org/10.1002/ptr.5858.

Arentz, Susan, et al. "Herbal Medicine for the Management of Polycystic Ovary Syndrome (PCOS) and Associated Oligo/Amenorrhoea and Hyperandrogenism; A Review of the Laboratory Evidence For Effects With Corroborative Clinical Findings" *BMC Complementary and Alternative Medicine* 14, no. 511 (December 2014): https://doi.org/10.1186/1472-6882-14-511.

Baumgartner, Christine et al. "Thyroid Function within the Normal Range, Subclinical Hypothyroidism, and the Risk of Atrial Fibrillation." *Circulation* 136, no. 22 (October 2017): 2100–16, https://doi.org/10.1161/CIRCULATIONAHA.117.028753.

Bronson, F. H. "Seasonal Variation in Human Reproduction: Environmental Factors." *Quarterly Review of Biology* 70, no. 2 (June 1995):141–64.

Boelen, Anita, Joan Kwakkel, and Eric Fliers. "Beyond Low Plasma T3: Local Thyroid Hormone Metabolism during Inflammation and Infection." *Endocrine Reviews* 32, no. 5 (October 2011): 670–93.

Bouayed, Jaouad, and Torsten Bohn. "Exogenous Antioxidants—Double-Edged Swords in Cellular Redox State: Health Beneficial Effects at Physiologic Doses versus Deleterious Effects at High Doses." *Oxidative Medicine and Cellular Longevity* 3, no. 4 (2010): 228–37, http://dx.doi.org/10.4161/oxim.3.4.12858.

Coppola, Anna, Rosaria Meli, and Sabrina Diano. "Inverse Shift in Circulating Corticosterone and Leptin Levels Elevates Hypothalamic Deiodinase Type 2 in Fasted Rats." *Endocrinology* 146, no. 6 (June 2005): 2827–33, https://doi.org/10.1210/en.2004-1361.

DeGroot, L. J. *The Non-Thyroidal Illness Syndrome*. [Updated February 1, 2015]. Edited by K. R. Feingold, B. Anawalt, A. Boyce, et al., Endotext [Internet]. South Dartmouth, MA: MDText.com, Inc.; 2000-. Available from https://www.ncbi.nlm.nih.gov/books/NBK285570/.

Duke Health. "Women with Low Cholesterol May be at Risk for Depression and Anxiety." Last modified January 20, 2016. https://corporate.dukehealth.org/news-listing/women-low-cholesterol-may-be-risk-depression-and-anxiety.

Durlinger, A L. et al. "Anti-Müllerian Hormone Attenuates the Effects of FSH on Follicle Development in the Mouse Ovary." *Endocrinology* 142, no. 11 (November 2001): 4891–99, https://doi.org/10.1210/endo.142.11.8486.

Garg, Deepika, and Reshef Tal. "The Role of AMH in the Pathophysiology of Polycystic Ovarian Syndrome." *Reproductive BioMedicine Online* 33, no. 1 (July 2016): 15–28, https://doi.org/10.1016/j.rbmo.2016.04.007.

Golombeck, S. G. "Nonthyroidal Illness Syndrome and Euthyroid Sick Syndrome in Intensive Care Patients." *Seminars in Perinatology* 32, no. 6 December 2008): 413–18, https://doi.org/10.1053/j.semperi.2008.09.010.

Grossman, Michael P., et al. "Müllerian-Inhibiting Substance Inhibits Cytochrome P450 Aromatase Activity in Human Granulosa Lutein Cell Culture." *Fertility and Sterility* 89, no. 5 (May 2008): 1364–70, https://doi.org/10.1016/j.fertnstert.2007.03.066.

Homburg, R. et al. "The Relationship of Serum Anti-Mullerian Hormone with Polycystic Ovarian Morphology and Polycystic Ovary Syndrome: A Prospective Cohort Study." *Human Reproduction* 28, no. 4 (February 2013): 1077–83, https://doi.org/10.1093/humrep/det015.

Jamil, Zehra, et al. "Assessment of Ovarian Reserve: Anti-Mullerian Hormone versus Follicle Stimulating Hormone." *Journal of Research in Medical Sciences* 21, no. 100 (November 2016): https://doi.org/10.4103/1735-1995.193172.

Johansson, Julia, and Elisabet Stener-Victorin. "Polycystic Ovary Syndrome: Effect and Mechanisms of Acupuncture for Ovulation Induction." *Evidence-Based Complementary and Alternative Medicine* 2013, no. 2013 (September 2013): 762615, https://doi.org/10.1155/2013/762615.

Lieberman, A., and L. Curtis. "In Defense of Progesterone: A Review of the Literature." *Alternative Therapies in Health and Medicine* 23, no. 6 (November 2017): 24–32.

Martinez, B., et. al. "Prolonged Food Deprivation Increases mRNA Expression of Deiodinase 1 and 2, and Thyroid Hormone Receptor β-1 in a Fasting-Adapted Mammal." *Journal of Experimental Biology* 216, no. 24 (December 2013): 4647–54, https://doi.org/10.1242/jeb.085290.

Ming, Jie et al. "Effectiveness and Safety of Bifidobacteria and Berberine in People with Hyperglycemia: Study Protocol for a Randomized Controlled Trial." *Trials* 19, no. 1 (January 2018): 72, https://doi.org/10.1186/s13063-018-2438-5.

Neto, Moura, Arnaldo, and Denise Engelbrecht Zantut-Wittmann. "Abnormalities of Thyroid Hormone Metabolism during Systemic Illness: The Low T3 Syndrome in Different Clinical Settings." *International Journal of Endocrinology* 2016 (2016): 2157583, http://dx.doi.org/10.1155/2016/2157583.

Nicoloff, J. T., Delbert A. Fisher, and Milo D. Appleman, Jr. "The Role of Glucocorticoids in the Regulation of Thyroid Function in Man." *Journal of Clinical Investigation* 49, no. 10 (October 1970): 1922–29, https://doi.org/10.1172/JCI106411.

Paoletti, J. "Differentiation and Treatment of Hypothyroidism, Functional Hypothyroidism, and Functional Metabolism." *International Journal of Pharmaceutical Compounding* 12, no. 6 (November/December 2008): 488–97.

Peeters R. P., and T. J. Visser. "Metabolism of Thyroid Hormone." [Updated January 1 2017]. Edited by K. R. Feingold, B. Anawalt, A. Boyce, et al., Endotext [Internet]. South Dartmouth, MA: MDText.com, Inc.; 2000-. Available from https://www.ncbi.nlm.nih.gov/books/NBK285570/.

Pergialiotis, V., et al. "Management of Endocrine Disease: The Impact Of Subclinical Hypothyroidism on Anthropometric Characteristics, Lipid, Glucose and Hormonal Profile of PCOS Patients: A Systematic Review and Meta-Analysis." *European Journal of Endocrinology* 176, no. 3 (2017): R159–66, https://doi.org/10.1530/EJE-16-0611.

Raja-Khan, Nazia, et al. "The Physiological Basis of Complementary and Alternative Medicines for Polycystic Ovary Syndrome." *American Journal of Physiology, Endocrinology and Metabolism* 301, no. 1 (July 2011): E1–10, https://doi.org/10.1152/ajpendo.00667.2010.

Rodriguez-Perez, Alfonso, et al. "Identification of Molecular Mechanisms Related to Nonthyroidal Illness Syndrome in Skeletal Muscle and Adipose Tissue from Patients with Septic Shock." *Clinical Endocrinology* 68, no. 5 (May 2008): 821–7, https://doi.org/10.1111/j.1365-2265.2007.03102.x.

Streuli, Isabelle et al. "Clinical Uses of Anti-Müllerian Hormone Assays: Pitfalls and Promises." *Fertility and Sterility* 91, no. 1 (January 2009): 226–30, https://doi.org/10.1016/j.fertnstert.2007.10.067.

Tibaldi, J. M., and M. I. Surks. "Effects of Nonthyroidal Illness on Thyroid Function." *Medical Clinics of North America* 69, no. 5 (September 1985): 899–911.

Zadehmodarres, Shahrzad, et al. "Anti-Mullerian Hormone Level and Polycystic Ovarian Syndrome Diagnosis." *Iranian Journal of Reproductive Medicine* 13, no. 4 (2015): 227–30.

Chapter 11

Abidov, M., et al. "Extract of *Rhodiola rosea radix* Reduces the Level of C-Reactive Protein and Creatinine Kinase in the Blood." *Pharmacology Biochemistry and Behavior* 138, no. 1 (July 2004): 63–4.

Boström, Pontus, et al. "A PGC1-α-Dependent Myokine That Drives Brown-Fat-Like Development of White Fat and Thermogenesis." *Nature* 481, no. 7382 (January 2012): 463–8, https://doi.org/10.1038/nature10777.

Bodinham, C. L., G. S. Frost, and M. D. Robertson "Acute Ingestion of Resistant Starch Reduces Food Intake in Healthy Adults." *British Journal of Nutrition* 103, no. 6 (March 2010): 917–22, https://doi.org/10.1017/S0007114509992534.

Chandrasekhar, K., Jyoti Kapoor, and Sridhar Anishetty. "A Prospective, Randomized Double-Blind, Placebo-Controlled Study of Safety and Efficacy of a High-Concentration Full-Spectrum Extract of Ashwagandha Root in Reducing Stress and Anxiety in Adults." *Journal of Psychological Medicine* 34, no. 3 (July 2012): 255–62, https://doi.org/10.4103/0253-7176.106022.

Chattopadhyay, D., et al. "A Potent Sperm Motility-Inhibiting Activity of Bioflavonoids from an Ethnomedicine of Onge, Alstonia macrophylla Wall ex A. DC, leaf extract." *Contraception* 71, no. 5 (May 2005): 372–8, https://doi.org/10.1016/j.contraception.2004.11.006.

De Souza, L. R., et al. "Korean Red Ginseng (*Panax ginseng* C.A. Meyer) Root Fractions: Differential Effects on Postprandial Glycemia In Healthy Individuals." *Journal of Ethnopharmacology* 137, no. 1 (September 2011): 245–50, https://doi.org/10.1016/j.jep.2011.05.015.

Forouhari, Sedighe, et al. "Effect of Vitamin C Supplementation on the Levels of Related Hormones in Infertile Women with Polycystic Ovary Syndrome (PCOS) in Shiraz City." *International Journal of Health Sciences* 2, no. 1, (March 2014): 61–70.

Halber, D. "Scientists Pinpoint Dosage of Melatonin for Insomnia." *MIT News,* October 17, 2001. http://news.mit.edu/2001/melatonin-1017.

Heid, Markam. "You Asked: Can Using a Laptop Make You Infertile?" *Time,* September 13, 2017. http://time.com/4938530/can-laptops-cause-infertility/.

Hongratanaworakit, T. "Aroma-Therapeutic Effects of Massage Blended Essential Oils on Humans." *Natural Product Communications* 6, no. 8 (August 2011): 1199–204.

Jahan, Sarwat et al. "Ameliorative Effects of Rutin against Metabolic, Biochemical and Hormonal Disturbances in Polycystic Ovary Syndrome in Rats." *Journal of Ovarian Research* 9, no. 1 (December 2016): 86, https://doi.org/10.1186/s13048-016-0295-y.

Jamshidi, Negar, and Marc M. Cohen. "The Clinical Efficacy and Safety of Tulsi in Humans: A Systematic Review of the Literature." *Evidence-Based Complementary and Alternative Medicine* 2017 (2017): 9217567, https://doi.org/10.1155/2017/9217567.

Khan, M. A., et al. "Effect of *Withania somnifera* (Ashwagandha) Root Extract on Amelioration of Oxidative Stress and Autoantibodies Production In Collagen-Induced Arthritic Rats." *Journal of Complementary and Integrative Medicine* 12, no. 2 (June 2015):117–25, https://doi.org/10.1515/jcim-2014-0075

Kıvrak, Elfide Gizem, et al. "Effects of Electromagnetic Fields Exposure on the Antioxidant Defense System." *Journal of Microscopy and Ultrastructure* 5, no. 4 (2017): 167–76, https://doi.org/10.1016/j.jmau.2017.07.003.

Koulivand, Peir Hossein, Maryam Khaleghi Ghadiri, and Ali Gorji. "Lavender and the Nervous System." *Evidence-Based Complementary and Alternative Medicine* 2013 (2013): 681304, https://doi.org/10.1155/2013/681304.

Kruse, Jack. n.d. "Can You Supplement Sunlight?" *Reversing Disease for Optimal Health*. Accessed April 17, 2019. https://jackkruse.com/time-10-can-you-supplement-sunlight/.

Leung, Tsz Wing, Roger Wing-hong Li, and Chea-su Kee. "Blue-Light Filtering Spectacle Lenses: Optical and Clinical Performances." *PloS One* 12, no. 1 (January 2017): e0169114, https://doi.org/10.1371/journal.pone.0169114.

Meissner, H. O., et al. "Hormone-Balancing Effect of Pre-Gelatinized Organic Maca (*Lepidium peruvianum* Chacon): (I) Biochemical and Pharmacodynamic Study on Maca Using Clinical Laboratory Model on Ovariectomized Rats." *International Journal of Biomedical Science*: 2, no. 3 (September 2006): 260–72.

Mora Murri, Manuel Luque-Ramírez, et al. "Circulating Markers of Oxidative Stress and Polycystic Ovary Syndrome (PCOS): A Systematic Review and Meta-Analysis." *Human Reproduction Update*, 19, no. 3 (May/June 2013): 268–88, https://doi.org/10.1093/humupd/dms059.

Panossian, Alexander, and Georg Wikman. "Effects of Adaptogens on the Central Nervous System and the Molecular Mechanisms Associated with Their Stress-Protective Activity." *Pharmaceuticals* 3, no. 1(January 2010): 188–224, https://doi.org/10.3390/ph3010188.

Rai, D. et al. "Adaptogenic Effect of *Bacopa monniera* (Brahmi)." *Pharmacology Biochemistry and Behavior* 75, no. 4 (July 2003): 823–30.

Rana, Digvijay G., and Varsha J, Galani. "Dopamine Mediated Antidepressant Effect of *Mucuna pruriens* Seeds in Various Experimental Models Of Depression."*Ayu* 35, no. 1 (2014): 90–7, https://doi.org/10.4103/0974-8520.141949.

Shukla, Kamla Kant, et al. "*Mucuna pruriens* Reduces Stress and Improves the Quality of Semen in Infertile Men." *Evidence-Based Complementary and Alternative Medicine* 7, no. 1 (2007): 137–44, https://doi.org/10.1093/ecam/nem171.

Song, J., et al. "Effect of Cs-4 (*Cordyceps sinensis*) on Exercise Performance in Healthy Older Subjects: A Double-Blind, Placebo-Controlled Trial." *Journal of Complementary and Integrative Medicine* 16, no. 5 (May 2010): 585–90, https://doi.org/10.1089/acm.2009.0226.

Tomaine. Gina. "I Wore Blue Light Blocking Glasses Every Day for a Week — Here's What I Learned." *Good Housekeeping,* July 11, 2018. https://www.goodhousekeeping.com/health/a20707076/blue-light-glasses/.

van Ballegooijen, Adriana J., et al. "The Synergistic Interplay between Vitamins D and K for Bone and Cardiovascular Health: A Narrative Review." *International Journal of Endocrinology* 2017 (2017): 7454376, https://doi.org/10.1155/2017/7454376.

Printed in Great Britain
by Amazon

41053716R00098